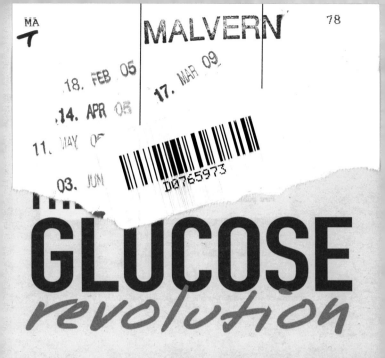

GLUCOSE
revolution

PROF JENNIE BRAND-MILLER
KAYE FOSTER-POWELL
DR SUSANNA HOLT

HODDER

First published in Great Britain in 2004 by Hodder and Stoughton
A division of Hodder Headline
This United Kingdom edition is published by arrangement with
Hodder Headline Australia Pty Limited

The right of Jennie Brand-Miller, Kaye Foster-Powell and Susanna Holt to be
identified as the Authors of the Work has been asserted by them in
accordance with the Copyright, Designs and Patents Act 1988

A Mobius Book

1 3 5 7 9 10 8 6 4 2

ISBN 0340835362

Typeset in Bembo

Printed and bound by Clays Ltd, St Ives plc

Hodder Headline's policy is to use papers that are natural, renewable and
recyclable products and made from wood grown in sustainable forests.
The logging and manufacturing processes are expected to conform
to the environmental regulations of the country of origin

Hodder and Stoughton Ltd
A division of Hodder Headline
338 Euston Road
London NW1 3BH

CONTENTS

INTRODUCTION

The GI values are the key to unlocking the enormous health benefits of *The New Glucose Revolution*.

People with diabetes, heart disease, the metabolic syndrome (Syndrome X) or people who are overweight will gain the most from putting *The New Glucose Revolution* approach into practice. But it's also for those who want to do the best they can to prevent those problems in the first place, and improve their overall health. In short, *The New Glucose Revolution* is for everybody.

With that in mind, we've put together this handy companion book full of GI values to help you put the GI into practice. There are three listings in this book:

- an A–Z list of individual foods for easy reference;
- a comprehensive list of foods and food categories for in-depth knowledge;
- and a simple food category list in GI value order for quick comparisons.

You can use the different listings to:

- find the GI of your favourite food
- compare foods within the same category (for instance, two types of bread) to see which is lower
- improve your diet by finding low GI substitutes for high GI foods
- find the lowest GI value within a food group easily
- compare the GI values of food groups
- put together a low GI meal
- shop for low GI foods
- check the GI value of products

If you can't find a GI value for a food you eat on many occasions, please write to the manufacturer and encourage them to have the GI of the food tested by an accredited laboratory such as Sydney University's Glycaemic Index Research Service (SUGiRS). In the meantime, use a similar food as a substitute.

In Australia the GI symbol (pictured on page 3) flags healthy foods that have been properly GI tested and includes their GI value on the packing. This type of labelling may be introduced in other countries in due course.

The GI values in this book are correct at the time of publication. However, the formulation of commercial foods can change and the GI may be altered. Check our webpage www.glycemicindex.com for the latest information.

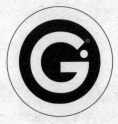

Footnote: Most testing of foods has been done in Australia, Canada and the USA. Products with identical brand names in the UK and Australia may differ slightly in composition and GI. These, and others which are not yet available in the UK, have not been deleted from the table as they give an approximate idea of the GI of similar UK products.

UNDERSTANDING THE GLYCAEMIC INDEX

Our research on the GI began in the 1980s when health authorities all over the world began to stress the importance of high carbohydrate diets. Until then dietary fat had grabbed all the public and scientific attention (and to some extent this is still true). But low fat diets are by their very nature *automatically* high in carbohydrate. Nutrition scientists started asking questions—are all carbohydrates the same, are all starches good for health, are all sugars bad? In particular, they began studies on the effects of carbohydrates on blood glucose levels. They wanted to know which carbohydrate foods were associated with the least fluctuation in blood glucose levels and the best overall health, including a reduced risk of diabetes and heart disease.

As we explain in our bestselling book, *The New Glucose Revolution*, the glycaemic index:

- is a scientifically proven measure of the effect carbohydrates have on blood glucose levels;
- helps you choose the right amount and type of carbohydrate for your health and wellbeing;
- provides an easy and effective way to eat a healthy diet and control fluctuations in blood glucose.

What is the GI

The GI is a physiologically based measure of carbohydrate quality—a comparison of carbohydrates (gram for gram) based on their immediate effects on blood glucose levels.

- Carbohydrates that break down quickly during digestion have high GI values. Their blood glucose response is fast and high.
- Carbohydrates that break down slowly, releasing glucose gradually into the bloodstream, have a low GI.

The rate of carbohydrate digestion has important implications for everybody. For most people, the foods with a low GI have advantages over those with high GI. This is especially true for people with diabetes or trying to control their weight.

A knowledge and appreciation of the GI will help you choose the right amount of carbohydrate and the right sort of carbohydrate for your lifestyle and well-being. We know from our own experience and letters from our readers that understanding the GI of foods makes an enormous difference to people's lives. For some it means a new lease of life.

For more detailed information about the GI, its effects and benefits, you should consult our other books, *The New Glucose Revolution* and *The New Glucose Revolution Life Plan*. These books also provide practical advice and tips about changing to low GI diets, improving your overall diet, foods to stock and buy, and delicious recipes to try.

LET'S TALK
GLYCAEMIC LOAD

As well as the GI values, the lists in this book include the glycaemic load (GL) value of average-sized portions of the foods to ensure you have all the information you need to choose foods which will improve your overall health.

Glycaemic load is the product of the GI and carbohydrate per serve of food. When we eat a meal containing carbohydrate, the blood glucose rises and falls. The extent to which it rises and remains high is critically important to health and depends on two things: the *amount* of a carbohydrate in the meal and the *nature* (GI) of that carbohydrate. Both are equally important determinants of changes in blood glucose levels.

Researchers at Harvard University came up with a way of combining and describing these two factors with the term 'glycaemic load'. It provides a measure of the degree of glycaemia and insulin demand produced by a normal serving of the food. GI values are measured for fixed portions of foods containing a certain amount of carbohydrate, usually 50 grams. However, as people eat different sized portions of the same foods, we can work out the extent to which a certain portion of food will raise the blood glucose level by calculating a glycaemic load value for that amount of food.

Glycaemic load is calculated simply by mulitplying the GI of a food by the amount of carbohydrate in that serving and dividing by 100.

$$\text{Glycaemic load} = (\text{GI} \times \text{carbohydrate per serving}) \div 100$$

For example, an apple has a GI of 40 and contains 15 grams of carbohydrate per serve. Its glycaemic load is $(40 \times 15) \div 100 = 6$. A potato has a GI of 90 and 20 grams of carbohydrate per serve. It has a glycaemic load of $(90 \times 20) \div 100 = 18$. This means one potato will raise your blood glucose level higher than one apple.

The glycaemic load is greatest for those foods which provide the most high GI carbohydrate, particularly those we tend to eat in large quantities. Compare the glycaemic load of the following foods to see how the serving size as well as the GI are significant in determining the glycaemic response:

Rice—1 cup of boiled white rice (150 g) contains 43 g carbohydrate and has a GI of 83. The glycaemic load is $(83 \times 43) \div 100 = 36$.

Spaghetti—1 serve (150 g) of cooked spaghetti contains 48 g carbohydrate and has a GI of 44. The glycaemic load is $(44 \times 48) \div 100 = 21$.

Some nutritionists have argued that the glycaemic load is an improvement on the GI because it provides an estimate of both quantity and quality of carbohydrate (the GI gives us just quality) in a diet. In large scale studies from Harvard University, however, the risk of disease was predicted by both the GI of the overall diet as well as the glycaemic load. The use of the glycaemic load strengthened the relationship, suggesting that the more frequent the consumption of high carbohydrate, high GI foods, the more adverse the health outcome. Carbohydrate by itself has no effect, ie there was no benefit of low carbohydrate intake over high carbohydrate intake, or vice versa.

Low GL = 10 or less
Intermediate GL = 11–19
High GL = 20 or more

Don't make the mistake of using GL alone. If you do, you might find yourself eating a diet with very little carbohydrate but a lot of fat, especially saturated fat, and excessive amounts of protein. Use the glycaemic index to compare foods of similar nature (eg bread with bread) and use the glycaemic load when comparing foods with a high GI but low carbohydrate content per serve (eg pumpkin).

Remember that the GL values listed are for the specified (nominal) portion size listed. If you eat a different portion size (ie weight), then you will need to calculate another GI value. First find out the weight of your portion, then work out the available carbohydrate content of this weight (this value is listed beside the GL) and then multiply by the food's GI value. For example, the nominal serve size listed for pumpkin is 80 grams, the available carbohydrate is 4 grams and the GI is 75. So the current GI is $(4 \times 75) \div 100 = 3$. If, however, you were eating twice the nominal size (160 grams, in this instance) you would need to double the available carbohydrate (8 grams, in this instance) and the GL for your larger serve of pumpkin would be: $(8 \times 75) \div 100 = 6$.

YOUR DAILY FOOD CHOICES

To guide your daily food choices we've created two GI food pyramids, one for moderate carbohydrate eaters and one for high carbohydrate eaters. The recommended servings of each food group are shown on each pyramid. If you are a big bread and cereal eater, the GI pyramid for high carbohydrate eaters will suit you best. Either way, the serving information on page 15 applies to both pyramids.

The base of the pyramid carries the text '60 minutes accumulated physical activity'. This is a reminder of the importance of exercise to overall health and well being.

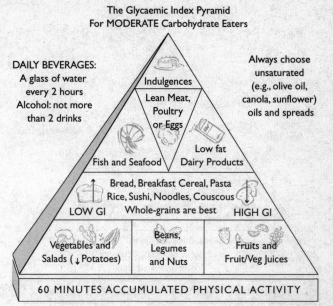

The Glycaemic Index Pyramid
For MODERATE Carbohydrate Eaters

DAILY BEVERAGES:
A glass of water
every 2 hours
Alcohol: not more
than 2 drinks

Always choose
unsaturated
(e.g., olive oil,
canola, sunflower)
oils and spreads

Indulgences

Lean Meat,
Poultry
or Eggs

Low fat
Dairy Products

Fish and Seafood

Bread, Breakfast Cereal, Pasta
Rice, Sushi, Noodles, Couscous
Whole-grains are best

LOW GI

HIGH GI

Vegetables and
Salads (↓ Potatoes)

Beans,
Legumes
and Nuts

Fruits and
Fruit/Veg Juices

60 MINUTES ACCUMULATED PHYSICAL ACTIVITY

DAILY

For moderate carbohydrate eaters:

Indulgences: 1–2 servings

Fish and seafood / Lean meat, poultry and eggs: 3–4 servings

Low fat dairy products: 3–4 servings

Bread, breakfast cereals, grains: 4–6 servings

Vegetables and salads: 4–6 servings

Beans, legumes and nuts: 1–2 serving

Fruits and juices: 2–3 servings

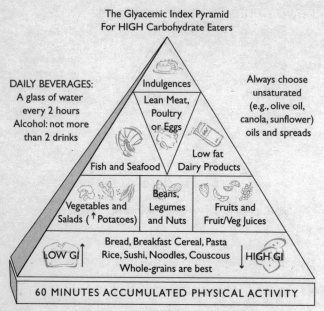

The Glyacemic Index Pyramid
For HIGH Carbohydrate Eaters

DAILY BEVERAGES:
A glass of water
every 2 hours
Alcohol: not more
than 2 drinks

Always choose
unsaturated
(e.g., olive oil,
canola, sunflower)
oils and spreads

Indulgences

Lean Meat,
Poultry
or Eggs

Low fat
Dairy Products

Fish and Seafood

Vegetables and
Salads (↑Potatoes)

Beans,
Legumes
and Nuts

Fruits and
Fruit/Veg Juices

LOW GI↑

Bread, Breakfast Cereal, Pasta
Rice, Sushi, Noodles, Couscous
Whole-grains are best

↓HIGH GI

60 MINUTES ACCUMULATED PHYSICAL ACTIVITY

DAILY

For high carbohydrate eaters:

Indulgences: 1–2 servings

Fish and seafood / Lean meat, poultry and eggs: 2–3 servings

Low fat dairy products: 2–3 servings

Bread, breakfast cereals, grains etc: 6–8 servings

Vegetables and salads: 4–6 servings

Beans, legumes and nuts: 1 serving

Fruits and juices: 3–4 servings

Serving information

The following answers the question of how much is a serve. The one set serves both pyramids.

INDULGENCES:
1 Tbsp (20 g) butter, margarine, oil
2 Tbsp (40 g) cream, mayonnaise
25 g chocolate
1 small slice (40 g) cake
1 small packet (30 g) potato crisps
2 standard alcoholic drinks alcohol

FISH AND SEAFOOD / LEAN MEAT, POULTRY AND EGGS:
80–120 g cooked fish
60–90 g cooked lean meat or poultry
1 egg

LOW FAT DAIRY PRODUCTS:
1 cup (250 ml) low fat milk or yoghurt
40 g reduced fat cheese

BREAD, BREAKFAST CEREALS, GRAINS ETC:
1 slice bread
30 g cereal
½ cup cooked rice, pasta or noodles

VEGETABLES & SALADS:

½ cup cooked vegetables

1 cup raw, salad vegetables

BEANS, LEGUMES AND NUTS:

1 cup cooked dried beans, peas or lentils

30 g nuts

FRUITS AND JUICES:

1 medium piece of fruit

1 cup of small fruit pieces

½ cup juice

A TO Z
GI VALUES

This is the place to go when you want to locate the GI value of a popular food quickly. Here foods are listed alphabetically—both on an individual basis and within their specific food category. For example, you will find Bürgen breads under both Breads and Bürgen. Food category entries include: biscuits, breads, breakfast cereal bars, breakfast cereals, cereal grains, crackers, dairy products, fruit, fruit juices, legumes, meat, pasta and noodles, potato, rice, snack foods, soft drinks, soups, sports drinks, sugars and honey, and vegetables.

We have also included some foods under their well-known brand or company names as well, for example Norco ice-cream appears as both 'Ice-cream (Norco)' and 'Norco Ice-cream'.

This a condensed listing of the GI values: we have given the average GI values for some foods. The average value may be calculated from the results of 10 separate studies of that food worldwide or only 2 to 4 studies. In a few instances, Australian data are different to the rest of the world and we show our data rather than the average. The food category listings on pages 48–104 are more comprehensive, showing the different studies and worldwide results.

In this listing you'll find not only the GI but the glycaemic load (GL = carbohydrate content × GI/100). The glycaemic load has been calculated using a 'nominal' serving size and the carbohydrate content of that serve, both of which are also listed. In this way, you can choose foods with either a low GI and/or a low GL. If your favourite food is both high GI and high GL, try to cut down the serving size or dilute the GL by teaming it with a very low GI food (eg rice and lentils).

We've also included some foods that contain very little carbohydrate and have therefore been automatically omitted from previous editions. However, so many people ask us for their GI, we decided the best thing was to include them and show their GI as [0]. Many vegetables such as avocadoes and broccoli, and protein-rich foods such as eggs, chicken, cheese and tuna are among the low or no carbohydrate category. Most alcoholic beverages are also low in carbohydrate. Beer has approximately 10 grams per middy, but its GI is unknown.

FOOD	GI	NOMINAL SERVE SIZE	AVAILABLE CARB PER SERVE	GL PER SERVE
All-Bran™, breakfast cereal	30	30 g	15	4
All-Bran Fruit 'n' Oats™, breakfast cereal	39	30 g	17	7
All-Bran Soy 'n' Fibre™, breakfast cereal	33	30 g	14	4
Angel food cake, 1 slice	67	50 g	29	19
Apple, raw, 1 medium	38*	120 g	15	6
Apple, dried	29	60 g	34	10
Apple juice, pure, unsweetened	40	250 ml	28	11
Apple muffin	44	60 g	29	13
Apple, oat and sultana muffin (from packet mix)	54	50 g	26	14
Apricots, raw, 3 medium	57	168 g	13	7
Apricots, canned in light syrup	64	120 g	19	12
Apricots, dried	30	60 g	27	8
Apricot, coconut and honey muffin (from mix)	60	50 g	26	16
Arborio, risotto rice, white, boiled	69	150 g	43	29
Bagel, white	72	70 g	35	25
Baked beans, canned in tomato sauce	48*	150 g	17	8
Banana, raw, 1 large	52*	120 g	26	13
Banana cake, 1 slice	47	80 g	38	18
Banana, oat and honey muffin (from packet mix)	65	50 g	26	17
Barley, pearled, boiled	25*	150 g	32	8
Basmati rice, white, boiled, 1 cup	58	150 g	42	24
Beef	[0]	120 g	0	0
Beer	[0]	250 ml	10 g	0
Beetroot, canned	64	80 g	7	5
Bengal gram dhal, chickpea	11	150 g	36	4
Biscuits				
Digestives	59*	25 g	16	10

* Average

FOOD	GI	NOMINAL SERVE SIZE	AVAILABLE CARB PER SERVE	GL PER SERVE
Highland Oatmeal™	55	25 g	18	10
Milk Arrowroot™	69	25 g	18	12
Morning Coffee™	79	25 g	19	15
Shortbread	64	25 g	16	10
Shredded Wheatmeal™	62	25 g	18	11
Snack Right™ Fruit Slice	48	25 g	19	9
Black bean soup	64	250 ml	27	17
Black beans, boiled	30	150 g	25	5
Blackbread (Riga)	76	30 g	13	10
Blackeyed beans, soaked, boiled	42	150 g	29	12
Blueberry muffin	59	57 g	29	17
Bran Flakes™, breakfast cereal	74	30 g	18	13
Bran muffin	60	57 g	24	15
Breads				
Bagel, white	72	70 g	35	25
Baguette, white	95	30 g	15	15
Barley flour bread	67	30 g	13	9
Blackbread (Riga)	76	30 g	13	10
Bürgen™ Oatbran and Honey	49	40 g	13	7
Bürgen™ Rye	51	40 g	13	7
Bürgen® Soy-Lin	36	30 g	9	3
Continental fruit loaf	47	30 g	15	7
Fruit and Spice Loaf (Buttercup)	54	30 g	15	8
Gluten-free multigrain bread	79	30 g	13	10
Hamburger bun, white	61	30 g	15	9
Helga's™ Classic Seed Loaf	68	30 g	14	9
Helga's™ traditional wholemeal bread	70	30 g	13	9
Hyfibre, white	70	67 g	27	19
Holsom's, sunflower and poppyseed	61	74 g	30	18

* Average

FOOD	GI	NOMINAL SERVE SIZE	AVAILABLE CARB PER SERVE	GL PER SERVE
Holsom's wholemeal and rye	63	74 g	28	18
Kaiser rolls	73	30 g	16	12
Lebanese bread, white	75	30 g	16	12
Melba toast	70	30 g	23	16
Multigrain Spelt wheat loaf	54	30 g	15	8
Multigrain (Tip Top)	65	30 g	28	18
9-Grain Multi-Grain (Tip-Top)	43	30 g	14	6
Pain au lait	63	60 g	32	20
Performax™ (Country Life)	38	30 g	13	5
Pita bread	57	30 g	17	10
Ploughman's™ Wholegrain	47	30 g	14	7
Ploughman's™ Wholemeal	64	30 g	13	9
Rice bread, high-amylose Doongara rice	61	30 g	12	7
Rice bread, low-amylose Calrose rice	72	30 g	12	8
Roggenbrot (Vogel's)	59	30 g	14	8
Schinkenbrot (Riga)	86	30 g	14	12
Sourdough rye	53*	30 g	12	6
Sourdough wheat	54	30 g	14	8
Spelt multigrain bread	54	30 g	12	7
Sunflower and barley bread (Riga)	57	30 g	11	6
Vogel's Honey & Oats	55	30 g	14	7
White bread	70	30 g	14	10
Wholemeal bread	77	30 g	12	9
Wholemeal rye bread	58*	30 g	14	8
Wonderwhite™ (Buttercup)	80	30 g	14	11
Breakfast cereal bars				
Crunchy Nut Cornflakes™ bar	72	30 g	26	19
Fibre Plus™ bar	78	30 g	23	18

* Average

FOOD	GI	NOMINAL SERVE SIZE	AVAILABLE CARB PER SERVE	GL PER SERVE
Fruity-Bix™ bar, fruit and nut	56	30 g	19	10
Fruity-Bix™ bar, wild berry	51	30 g	19	9
K-Time Just Right™ bar	72	30 g	24	17
K-Time Strawberry Crunch™ bar	77	30 g	25	19
Rice Bubble Treat™ bar	63	30 g	24	15
Sustain™ bar	57	30 g	25	14
Breakfast cereals				
All-Bran™	30	30 g	15	5
All-Bran Fruit 'n' Oats™	39	30 g	17	7
All-Bran Soy 'n' Fibre™	33	30 g	14	4
Bran Flakes™	74	30 g	18	13
Coco Pops™	77	30 g	26	20
Cornflakes™	77	30 g	25	20
Cornflakes, Crunchy Nut™	72	30 g	24	17
Corn Pops™	80	30 g	26	21
Froot Loops™	69	30 g	26	18
Frosties™	55	30 g	26	15
Golden Wheats™	71	30 g	23	16
Good Start™, muesli wheat biscuits	68	30 g	20	14
Guardian™	37	30 g	12	5
Healthwise™ for bowel health	66	30 g	18	12
Healthwise™ for heart health	48	30 g	19	9
Hi-Bran Weet-Bix™	61	30 g	17	10
Hi-Bran Weet-Bix™ with soy and linseed	57	30 g	16	9
Hyfibre, white sandwich bread	70	67 g	27	19
Holsom's sunflower and poppyseed bread	61	74 g	30	18

* Average

FOOD	GI	NOMINAL SERVE SIZE	AVAILABLE CARB PER SERVE	GL PER SERVE
Holsom's wholemeal and rye bread	63	74 g	28	18
Honey Goldies™	72	30 g	21	15
Honey Rice Bubbles™	77	30 g	27	20
Honey Smacks™	71	30 g	23	16
Just Right™	60	30 g	22	13
Just Right Just Grains™	62	30 g	23	14
Komplete™	48	30 g	21	10
Lite-Bix™, no added sugar	70	30 g	20	14
Mini Wheats™, whole wheat	58	30 g	21	12
Mini Wheats™, blackcurrant	72	30 g	21	15
Muesli, gluten-free	39	30 g	19	7
Muesli, Natural	48*	30 g	18	8
Muesli, toasted (Purina)	43	30 g	17	7
Nutrigrain™	66	30 g	15	10
Oat 'n' Honey Bake™	77	30 g	17	13
Oat bran Weet-Bix™	57	30 g	20	11
Porridge, made from whole rolled oats	55*	250 g	21	11
Porridge, traditional oats	51	250 g	21	11
Porridge, instant	66*	250 g	26	17
Pop Tarts™, chocolate	70	50 g	36	25
Puffed Wheat	80	30 g	21	17
Rice Bran, extruded (Rice Growers)	19	30 g	14	3
Rice Bubbles™	87	30 g	26	22
Shredded Wheat	75	30 g	20	15
Soy Tasty™	60	30 g	20	12
Soytana™ (Vogel's)	49	45 g	25	12
Special K™	54	30 g	21	11
Sultana Bran™	73	30 g	19	14

* Average

FOOD	GI	NOMINAL SERVE SIZE	AVAILABLE CARB PER SERVE	GL PER SERVE
Sultana Goldies™	65	30 g	21	13
Sustain™	68	30 g	22	15
Ultra-bran™, soy and linseed	41	30 g	13	5
Vita-Brits™	68	30 g	20	13
Wheat-bites™	72	30 g	25	18
Weet-Bix™	69	30 g	17	12
Whole wheat Goldies™	70	30 g	20	14
Breton™ wheat crackers	67	25 g	14	10
Broad beans	79	80 g	11	9
Broken rice, white, cooked in rice cooker	86	150 g	43	37
Buckwheat, boiled	54*	150 g	30	16
Buckwheat, pancakes, gluten-free, made from packet mix	102	77 g	22	22
Bulghur, boiled 20 min	48*	150 g	26	12
Bun, hamburger	61	30 g	15	9
Bürgen® Oat Bran & Honey	49	40 g	13	7
Bürgen® Soy-Lin, kibbled soy (8%) and linseed (8%) loaf	36	30 g	9	3
Bürgen® Fruit Loaf	44	30 g	13	6
Bürgen® Mixed Grain	49*	30 g	11	6
Burger Rings™, barbeque-flavoured	90	50 g	31	28
Butter beans, dried, boiled	31*	150 g	20	6
Calrose rice, white, medium grain, boiled	83	150 g	42	35
Capellini pasta, boiled	45	180 g	45	20
Capsicum	[0]	80 g	0	0
Carrots, peeled, boiled	41*	80 g	5	2
Cereal grains				
Arborio, risotto rice, boiled	69	150 g	53	36
Barley, rolled, dry	66	50 g	38	25

* Average

FOOD	GI	NOMINAL SERVE SIZE	AVAILABLE CARB PER SERVE	GL PER SERVE
Basmati rice, boiled, white (Mahatma, Australia)	58	150 g	38	22
Buckwheat, boiled	54	150 g	30	16
Calrose rice, brown, boiled	87	150 g	38	33
Calrose rice, white, medium grain, boiled	83	150 g	43	36
Cornmeal, boiled	69	150 g	13	9
Corn, sweet	48	150 g	30	14
Couscous	65	150 g	33	21
Cracked wheat (bulghur), cooked	48*	150 g	26	12
Doongara rice, brown, boiled	66	150 g	37	24
Doongara rice, white	56	150 g	39	22
Instant rice, white, cooked 6 min	87	150 g	42	36
Instant Doongara rice, white	94	150 g	42	35
Koshikari (Japanese) white rice, boiled	48	150 g	42	20
Jasmine rice	109	150 g	42	46
Long grain rice, boiled	56	150 g	41	23
Parboiled, Doongara rice, boiled	50	150 g	39	19
Parboiled rice, Sungold	87	150 g	39	34
Pearl Barley, boiled	25	150 g	32	8
Pelde rice, brown, boiled	76	150 g	38	29
Pelde rice, white	93	150 g	43	40
Rice, brown, boiled	55	150 g	33	18
Rice, boiled, white	56	150 g	42	23
Rye, whole kernels, cooked	34	50 g	38	13
Semolina, cooked	55	150 g	11	6
Sunbrown rice, Quick™, boiled	80	150 g	38	31
Sungold rice, Pelde, parboiled	87	150 g	43	37
Wheat, whole kernels, cooked	41	50 g	34	14
Wheat, quick-cooking kernels	54	150 g	47	25

* Average

FOOD	GI	NOMINAL SERVE SIZE	AVAILABLE CARB PER SERVE	GL PER SERVE
Cheese	[0]	120 g	0	0
Cherries, raw	22	120 g	12	3
Chickpeas, canned in brine	42	150 g	22	9
Chickpeas, dried, boiled	28*	150 g	24	7
Chicken nuggets, frozen, reheated in microwave oven 5 min	46	100 g	16	7
Chocolate, plain, milk	43*	50 g	28	12
Chocolate, white, Milky Bar®	44	50 g	29	13
Chocolate butterscotch muffins, made from packet mix	53	50 g	28	15
Chocolate cake made from packet mix with chocolate frosting	38	111 g	52	20
Chocolate mousse, 2% fat	31	50 g	11	3
Chocolate pudding, instant made from packet with whole milk	47	100 g	16	7
Coca Cola®, soft drink	53	250 ml	26	14
Coco Pops™	77	30 g	26	20
Condensed milk, sweetened, full-fat	61	50 ml	28	17
Cordial, orange, reconstituted	66	250 ml	20	13
Corn chips, plain, salted	42	50 g	25	11
Cornflakes™, breakfast cereal	77	30 g	25	20
Cornflakes Crunchy Nut™, breakfast cereal	72	30 g	24	17
Cornmeal, boiled in salted water 2 min	68	150 g	13	9
Corn pasta, gluten-free, boiled	78	180 g	42	32
Corn Pops™, breakfast cereal	80	30 g	26	21
Corn Thins, puffed corn cakes, gluten-free	87	25 g	20	18
Couscous, boiled 5 min	65*	150 g	33	21
Crackers				
Breton wheat crackers	67	25 g	14	10

* Average

FOOD	GI	NOMINAL SERVE SIZE	AVAILABLE CARB PER SERVE	GL PER SERVE
Jatz™, plain salted crackers	55	25 g	17	10
Kavli™ Norwegian Crispbread	71	25 g	16	12
Puffed Crispbread	81	25 g	19	15
Puffed rice cakes	82	25 g	21	17
Rye crispbread	64	25 g	16	11
Sao™, plain square crackers	70	25 g	17	12
Vita-wheat™, original, crispbread	55	25 g	19	10
Water cracker	78	25 g	18	14
Cranberry juice cocktail	52	250 ml	31	16
Crispix™, breakfast cereal	87	30 g	25	22
Croissant	67	57 g	26	17
Crumpet, white	69	50 g	19	13
Crunchy Nut Cornflakes™ bar	72	30 g	26	19
Crunchy Nut™ Cornflakes	72	30 g	24	17
Cupcake, strawberry-iced	73	38 g	26	19
Custard, home made from milk, (wheat starch), and sugar	43	100 ml	17	7
Custard, prepared from powder with whole milk, No Bake™ (Nestlé)	35	100 ml	17	6
Custard, TRIM™, reduced-fat	37	100 ml	15	6
Custard apple, raw, flesh only	54	120 g	19	10
Dairy products				
Custard	38*	100 ml	16	6
Ice-cream, reduced	61	50 g	13	8
Peter's Light Ice-cream, vanilla, low-fat	50	50 g	6	3
Ice-cream, vanilla Prestige Light™ (Norco, Australia)	47	50 g	10	5
Ice-cream, Prestige Light™ traditional toffee (Norco, Australia)	37	50 g	14	5

* Average

FOOD	GI	NOMINAL SERVE SIZE	AVAILABLE CARB PER SERVE	GL PER SERVE
Ice-cream, Prestige™, golden macadamia (Norco, Australia)	37	50 g	9	3
Ice-cream, Premium Ultra chocolate, 15% fat (Sara Lee, Australia)	37	50 g	9	4
Ice-cream, French vanilla, 16% fat (Sara Lee, Australia)	38	50 g	9	3
Milk, full-fat, fresh	31	250 ml	12	4
Milk, low fat, chocolate, no added sugar	24	250 ml	15	3
Milk, chocolate, sugar-sweetened	43	50 ml	28	12
Mousse, reduced fat, from mix	34*	50 g	10	4
Peter's light & creamy™ vanilla ice-cream	44	50 g	13	6
Yoghurt, low fat, fruit, aspartame, Ski™	14	200 ml	13	2
Low fat, fruit, sugar, Ski™	33	200 ml	31	10
Yoghurt, no-fat, French vanilla, Vaalia, with sugar	40	150 ml	27	10
Yoghurt, no-fat, Mango, Vaalia, with sugar	39	150 ml	25	10
Yoghurt, no-fat, Wildberry, Vaalia, with sugar	38	150 ml	22	8
Yoghurt, no-fat, Strawberry, Vaalia, with sugar	38	150 ml	22	8
Yoghurt drink, Reduced-fat Vaalia™, passionfruit	38	200 ml	29	11
Dark rye, Blackbread (Riga)	76	30 g	13	10
Dark rye, Schinkenbrot (Riga)	86	30 g	14	12
Dates, dried	103	60 g	40	42
Desiree potato, peeled, boiled 35 min	101	150 g	17	17
Dietworks™ Hazelnut & Apricot bar	42	50 g	22	9

* Average

FOOD	GI	NOMINAL SERVE SIZE	AVAILABLE CARB PER SERVE	GL PER SERVE
Digestives plain, 2 biscuits	59*	25 g	16	10
Doongara, rice, white, boiled	56*	150 g	42	24
Egg Custard, prepared from powdered mix with whole milk, no bake	35	100 ml	17	6
Eggs	[0]	120 g	0	0
Ensure™, vanilla drink	48	250 ml	34	16
Ensure™ bar, chocolate fudge brownie	43	38 g	20	8
Ensure Plus™, vanilla drink	40	237 ml	40	19
Ensure Pudding™, old-fashioned vanilla	36	113 g	26	9
Fanta®, orange soft drink	68	250 ml	34	23
Fettuccine, egg, cooked	32	180 g	46	15
Figs, dried, tenderised	61	60 g	26	16
Fish	[0]	120 g	0	0
Fish fillet, crumbed (Maggi)	43	85 g	16	7
Fish Fingers	38	100 g	19	7
French baguette, white, plain	95	30 g	15	15
French fries, frozen, reheated in microwave	75	150 g	29	22
French vanilla ice-cream, premium, 16% fat (Sara Lee)	38	50 g	9	3
Froot Loops™, breakfast cereal	69	30 g	26	18
Frosties™, sugar-coated Cornflakes	55	30 g	26	15
Fructose, pure	19*	10 g	10	2
Vanilla cake made from packet mix with vanilla frosting	42	111 g	58	24
Fruit				
Apple	38*	120 g	15	6
Apple, dried	29	60 g	34	10
Apricots, dried	31*	60 g	28	9

* Average

FOOD	GI	NOMINAL SERVE SIZE	AVAILABLE CARB PER SERVE	GL PER SERVE
Banana	52*	120 g	26	13
Cherries	22	120 g	12	3
Dates, dried	103	60 g	40	42
Figs, dried	61	60 g	26	16
Grapefruit	25	120 g	11	3
Grapes, raw	46*	120 g	18	8
Grapes, black	59	120 g	18	11
Kiwi fruit	53*	120 g	12	6
Lychee, canned in syrup, drained	79	120 g	20	16
Mango	51*	120 g	17	8
Oranges	42*	120 g	11	5
Paw paw	59*	120 g	8	5
Peach	42*	120 g	11	5
Peach, canned in natural juice	38	120 g	11	4
Pears	38*	120 g	11	4
Pear halves, canned in reduced-sugar syrup, (SPC Lite)	25	120 g	14	4
Pear halves, canned in natural juice (SPC)	43	120 g	13	5
Pineapple, raw	59*	120 g	13	7
Plum, raw	39*	120 g	12	5
Prunes, pitted (Sunsweet)	29	60 g	33	10
Raisins	64	60 g	44	28
Rockmelon	65	120 g	6	4
Strawberries	40	120 g	3	1
Sultanas	56	60 g	45	25
Watermelon, raw	72	120 g	6	4
Fruit cocktail, canned	55	120 g	16	9
Fruit Fingers, Heinz Kidz™, banana	61	30 g	20	12
Fruit Juices				
Apple juice, unsweetened	40	250 ml	29	12

* Average

FOOD	GI	NOMINAL SERVE SIZE	AVAILABLE CARB PER SERVE	GL PER SERVE
Apple juice, pure, clear (Wild About Fruit, Australia)	44	250 ml	30	13
Apple juice, pure, cloudy (Wild About Fruit, Australia)	37	250 ml	28	10
Carrot juice, fresh	43	250 ml	23	10
Cranberry juice cocktail	52	250 ml	31	16
Grapefruit juice, unsweetened	48	250 ml	22	11
Orange juice, unsweetened	50*	250 ml	19	9
Pineapple juice, unsweetened	46	250 ml	34	16
Tomato juice, canned, no added sugar	38	250 ml	9	4
Fruit loaf, Bürgen™	44	30 g	13	6
Fruit Loaf, dense continental style wheat bread with dried fruit	47	30 g	15	7
Fruit and Spice Loaf, thick sliced	54	30 g	15	8
Gatorade® sports drink	78	250 ml	15	12
Glucodin™ glucose tablets	102	10 g	10	10
Gluten-free white bread, sliced	80	30 g	15	12
Gluten-free multigrain bread	79	30 g	13	10
Gluten-free muesli, with 1.5% fat milk	39	30 g	19	7
Gluten-free corn pasta	78	180 g	42	32
Gluten-free rice and maize pasta	76	180 g	49	37
Gluten-free split pea and soy pasta shells	29	180 g	31	9
Gluten-free spaghetti, rice and split pea, canned in tomato sauce	68	220 g	27	19
Glutinous rice, white, cooked in rice cooker	98	150 g	32	31
Gnocchi, cooked (Latina)	68	180 g	48	33
Golden Wheats™, breakfast cereal	71	30 g	23	16
Grapefruit, raw	25	120 g	11	3
Grapefruit juice, unsweetened	48	250 ml	20	9

* Average

FOOD	GI	NOMINAL SERVE SIZE	AVAILABLE CARB PER SERVE	GL PER SERVE
Grapes, green	46*	120 g	18	8
Green pea soup, canned	66	250 ml	41	27
Guardian™, breakfast cereal	37	30 g	12	5
Hamburger bun	61	30 g	15	9
Haricot/navy beans, cooked/canned	38*	150 g	31	12
Healthwise™ breakfast cereal for bowel health	66	30 g	18	12
Healthwise™ breakfast cereal for heart health	48	30 g	19	9
Helga's™ Classic Seed Loaf	68	30 g	14	9
Helga's™ traditional wholemeal bread	70	30 g	13	9
Honey, Yellow Box honey	35	25 g	18	6
Honey, Stringybark	44	25 g	21	9
Honey, Ironbark	48	25 g	15	7
Honey, Capilano	64*	25 g	17	11
Honey & Oat bread, Vogel's	55	30 g	14	7
Honey Rice Bubbles™, breakfast cereal	77	30 g	27	20
Honey Smacks™, breakfast cereal	71	30 g	23	11
Ice-cream, Norco, Prestige Light rich Vanilla	47	50 g	10	5
Ice-cream, Norco, Prestige Light Toffee	37	50 g	14	5
Ice-cream, Norco, Prestige Macadamia	39	50 g	12	5
Ice-cream, regular, average	61*	50 g	13	8
Ice-cream, Peter's light and creamy	44	100 ml	14	6
Ice-cream, premium, French vanilla, 16% fat	38	50 g	9	3
Ice-cream, premium, 'ultra chocolate', 15% fat	37	50 g	9	4
Instant mashed potato, prepared	69*	150 g	20	17

* Average

FOOD	GI	NOMINAL SERVE SIZE	AVAILABLE CARB PER SERVE	GL PER SERVE
Instant rice, white, cooked 6 min	87	150 g	42	29
Ironman PR bar®, chocolate	39	65 g	26	10
Isostar® sports drink	70	250 ml	18	13
Jam, apricot fruit spread, reduced sugar	55	30 g	13	7
Jam, strawberry, regular	51	30 g	20	10
Jasmine rice, white, long-grain, cooked in rice cooker	109	150 g	42	46
Jatz™, plain salted cracker biscuits	55	25 g	17	10
Jelly Beans	78*	30 g	28	22
Jevity™, fibre-enriched drink	48	237 ml	36	17
Just Right™, breakfast cereal	60	30 g	22	13
Just Right Just Grains™, breakfast cereal	62	30 g	23	14
Kaiser rolls	73	30 g	16	12
Kavli™ Norwegian Crispbread	71	25 g	16	12
Kidney beans, canned	52	150 g	17	9
Kidz™, Heinz, Fruit Fingers, banana	61	30 g	20	12
Kidney beans, boiled	28*	150 g	25	7
Kiwi fruit, raw	58	120 g	12	7
Komplete™, breakfast cereal	48	30 g	21	10
K-Time Just Right™ breakfast cereal bar	72	30 g	24	17
K-Time Strawberry Crunch™ breakfast cereal bar	77	30 g	25	19
Lactose, pure	46*	10 g	10	5
Lamb	[0]	120 g	0	0
Lamingtons, sponge dipped in chocolate and coconut	87	50 g	29	25
L.E.A.N Fibergy™ bar, Harvest Oat	45	50 g	29	13
L.E.A.N Life long Nutribar™, Peanut Crunch	30	40 g	19	6

* Average

33

FOOD	GI	NOMINAL SERVE SIZE	AVAILABLE CARB PER SERVE	GL PER SERVE
L.E.A.N Life long Nutribar™, Chocolate Crunch	32	40 g	19	6
L.E.A.N Nutrimeal™, drink powder, Dutch Chocolate	26	250 g	13	3
Lebanese bread, white, 1 round	75	83 g	45	34
Legumes				
Baked Beans, canned	48*	150 g	17	8
Blackeyed beans, boiled	42*	150 g	21	12
Butter Beans	31	150 g	20	6
Chickpeas, dried, boiled	28*	150 g	24	7
Haricot/navy beans, dried, cooked	38	150 g	31	12
Kidney beans	28	150 g	25	7
Lentils, boiled	29*	150 g	18	5
Lentils, green, dried, boiled	30*	150 g	17	5
Lentils, red, dried, boiled	26*	150 g	18	5
Lima beans	32	150 g	30	10
Marrowfat peas, dried, boiled	39*	150 g	19	7
Mung bean, dried, boiled	31	150 g	17	5
Peas, dried, boiled	22	150 g	9	2
Soy beans, dried, boiled	18*	150 g	6	1
Split peas, yellow, boiled	32	150 g	19	6
Lentils, canned, green	52	50 g	17	9
Lentils, green, dried, boiled	30*	150 g	17	5
Lentils, boiled	29*	150 g	18	5
Lentils, red, boiled	26	150 g	18	5
Life Savers®, peppermint	70	30 g	30	21
Light rye bread	68	30 g	14	10
Lima beans, baby, frozen, reheated in microwave oven	32	150 g	30	10
Linguine pasta, thick, cooked	46*	180 g	48	22
Linguine pasta, thin, cooked	52*	180 g	45	23

* Average

FOOD	GI	NOMINAL SERVE SIZE	AVAILABLE CARB PER SERVE	GL PER SERVE
Lucozade®, original, sparkling glucose drink	95	250 ml	42	40
Lungkow beanthread noodles	26	180 g	45	12
Lychees, canned in syrup, drained	79	120 g	20	16
M & M's®, peanut	33	30 g	17	6
Macaroni, plain, boiled	47*	180 g	48	23
Macaroni and Cheese, made from mix	64	180 g	51	32
Maltose, 50 g	105	10 g	10	11
Mango raw	51*	120 g	17	8
Maple syrup, Pure Canadian	54	24 g	18	10
Marmalade, orange	48	30 g	20	9
Mars Bar®	62	60 g	40	25
Meat				
Beef	[0]	120 g	0	0
Lamb	[0]	120 g	0	0
Pork	[0]	120 g	0	0
Salami	[0]	120 g	0	0
Tuna	[0]	120 g	0	0
Veal	[0]	120 g	0	0
Melba toast	70	30 g	23	16
Milk, full-fat cow's milk, fresh	31	250 ml	12	4
Milk, skim	32	250 ml	13	4
Milk, low fat, chocolate, with sugar, Lite White™	34	250 ml	26	9
Milk, condensed, sweetened	61	50 ml	28	17
Milk Arrowroot™ biscuits	69	25 g	18	12
Milky Bar®, plain, white chocolate	44	50 g	29	13
Millet, boiled	71	150 g	36	25
Milo™, chocolate powder, dissolved in water	54	250 ml	16	9

* Average

FOOD	GI	NOMINAL SERVE SIZE	AVAILABLE CARB PER SERVE	GL PER SERVE
Milo™, ready to drink bottle	30	600 ml	66	20
Mini Wheats™, whole wheat breakfast cereal	58	30 g	21	12
Mini Wheats™, blackcurrant whole wheat breakfast cereal	72	30 g	21	15
Mixed grain loaf, Bürgen®	49*	30 g	11	6
Morning Coffee™, 3 biscuits	79	25 g	19	15
Mousse, butterscotch, reduced fat	36	50 g	10	4
Mousse, chocolate, reduced fat	31	50 g	11	3
Mousse, hazelnut, reduced fat	36	50 g	10	4
Mousse, mango, reduced fat	33	50 g	11	4
Mousse, mixed berry, reduced fat	36	50 g	10	4
Mousse, strawberry, reduced fat	32	50 g	10	3
Muesli bar containing dried fruit	61	30 g	21	13
Muesli, gluten-free with 1.5% fat milk	39	30 g	19	7
Muesli, toasted (Purina)	43	30 g	17	7
Muesli, Swiss Formula, natural	56	30 g	16	9
Multi-Grain 9-Grain	43	30 g	14	6
Mung bean noodles (Lungkow beanthread), dried, boiled	39	180 g	45	18
Nesquik™ powder, chocolate dissolved in 1.5% fat milk	41	250 ml	11	5
Nesquik™ powder, strawberry dissolved in 1.5% fat milk	35	250 ml	12	4
New potato, unpeeled and boiled 20 min	78	150 g	21	16
New potato, canned, heated in microwave 3 min	65	150 g	18	12
No Bake Egg Custard, prepared from powder with whole milk	35	100 ml	17	6
Noodles, instant 'two-minute' Maggi®	47*	180 g	40	19

* Average

FOOD	GI	NOMINAL SERVE SIZE	AVAILABLE CARB PER SERVE	GL PER SERVE
Noodles, mung bean (Lungkow beanthread), dried, boiled	39	180 g	45	18
Noodles, rice, freshly made, boiled	40	180 g	39	15
Norco Ice-cream, Prestige Light rich Vanilla	47	50 g	10	5
Norco Ice-cream, Prestige Light Toffee	37	50 g	14	5
Norco Ice-cream, Prestige Macadamia	39	50 g	12	5
Nutella®, chocolate hazelnut spread	33	20 g	12	4
Nutrigrain™, breakfast cereal	66	30 g	15	10
Oat 'n' Honey Bake™, breakfast cereal	77	30 g	17	13
Oat Bran & Honey Loaf bread, Bürgen®	49	40 g	13	7
Oat bran, raw	55*	10 g	5	3
Orange, 1 medium	42*	120 g	11	5
Orange cordial, reconstituted	66	250 ml	20	13
Orange juice, unsweetened, reconstituted	53	250 ml	18	9
Pancakes, prepared from shake mix	67	70 g	23	15
Pancakes, buckwheat, gluten-free, made from packet mix	102	77 g	22	22
Parsnips	97	80 g	12	12
Party pies, beef, cooked	45	100 g	27	12
Pasta and noodles				
Fettucine, egg, boiled	40*	180 g	46	18
Gnocchi	68	180 g	48	33
Instant noodles	47*	180 g	40	19
Linguine	49*	180 g	47	23
Mung bean noodles	39	180 g	45	18
Macaroni	47	180 g	48	23
Macaroni and Cheese, boxed	64	180 g	51	32

* Average

FOOD	GI	NOMINAL SERVE SIZE	AVAILABLE CARB PER SERVE	GL PER SERVE
Ravioli, meat-filled	39	180 g	38	15
Rice noodles, freshly made	40	180 g	39	15
Rice noodles, dried, boiled	61	180 g	39	23
Rice pasta, brown boiled	92	180 g	38	35
Spaghetti, gluten-free, canned in tomato sauce	68	220 g	27	19
Spaghetti, white, boiled 10-15 min	44*	180 g	48	21
Spaghetti, white, boiled 20 min	61*	180 g	44	27
Spaghetti, white, boiled	42*	180 g	47	20
Spaghetti, wholemeal, boiled	37*	180 g	42	16
Spirali, durum wheat, white, boiled	43	180 g	44	19
Udon noodles, plain	62	180 g	48	30
Pastry, plain	59	57 g	26	15
Paw paw, raw	59*	120 g	8	5
Peach, fresh, 1 large	42*	120 g	11	5
Peach, canned in heavy syrup	58	120 g	15	9
Peach, canned in light syrup	52	120 g	18	9
Peach, canned in reduced-sugar syrup, SPC Lite	62	120 g	17	11
Peanuts, roasted, salted	14*	50 g	6	1
Pear, raw	38*	120 g	11	4
Pear halves, canned in natural juice	43	120 g	13	5
Pear halves, canned in reduced-sugar syrup, (SPC Lite)	25	120 g	14	4
Peas, dried, boiled	22	150 g	9	2
Peas, green, frozen, boiled	48*	80 g	7	3
Pecans (raw)	10	50 g	3	1
Pelde brown rice, boiled	76	150 g	38	29
Performax™ bread	38	30 g	13	5

* Average

FOOD	GI	NOMINAL SERVE SIZE	AVAILABLE CARB PER SERVE	GL PER SERVE
Pikelets, Golden brand	85	40 g	21	18
Pineapple, raw	59*	120 g	10	6
Pineapple juice, unsweetened	46	250 ml	34	15
Pinto beans, canned in brine	45	150 g	22	10
Pinto beans, dried, boiled	39	150 g	26	10
Pita bread, white	57	30 g	17	10
Pizza, cheese	60	100 g	27	16
Pizza, Super Supreme, pan (11.4% fat)	36	100 g	24	9
Pizza, Super Supreme, thin and crispy (13.2 % fat)	30	100 g	22	7
Ploughman's™ Wholegrain bread, original recipe	47	30 g	14	7
Ploughman's™ Wholemeal bread, smooth milled	64	30 g	13	9
Plums, raw	39*	120 g	12	5
Pontiac potato, peeled, boiled 35 min	88	150 g	18	16
Pontiac potato, peeled and microwave on high for 6–7.5 min	79	150 g	18	14
Pontiac potato, peeled, cubed, boiled 15 min, mashed	91	150 g	20	18
Pop Tarts™, Double Chocolate	70	50 g	36	25
Popcorn, plain, cooked in microwave oven	72*	20 g	11	8
Pork	[0]	120 g	0	0
Porridge made from whole oats	55	250 g	21	12
Potato				
Baked potato, Ontario, with skin	60	150 g	30	18
Baked without fat Russet Burbank potato	85*	150 g	30	26
Canned potato, new	65	150 g	18	12
Desiree, peeled, boiled 35 min	101	150 g	17	17
French fries	75	150 g	29	22

* Average

FOOD	GI	NOMINAL SERVE SIZE	AVAILABLE CARB PER SERVE	GL PER SERVE
Instant mashed potato	85	150 g	20	17
New potato	62	150 g	21	13
Ontario, peeled, boiled 35 min	58	150 g	27	16
Pontiac, peeled, boiled 35 min	88	150 g	18	16
Mashed potato				
Pontiac, mashed	91	150 g	20	18
Pontiac, peeled and microwaved on high for 6–7.5 min	79	150 g	18	14
Potato, peeled, steamed	65	150 g	27	18
Sebago, peeled, boiled 35 min	87	150 g	17	14
Sweet potato	44	150 g	25	11
Potato crisps, plain, salted	54*	50 g	21	11
Pound cake	54	53 g	28	15
Power Bar®, chocolate	56*	65 g	42	24
Pretzels, oven-baked, traditional wheat flavour	83	30 g	20	16
Prunes, pitted, 6	29	60 g	33	10
Pudding, instant, chocolate, made from powder and whole milk	47	100 g	16	7
Pudding, instant, vanilla, made from powder and whole milk	40	100 g	16	6
Pudding, Sustagen™, instant vanilla, made from powdered mix	27	250 g	47	13
Puffed crispbread	81	25 g	19	15
Puffed rice cakes, white	82	25 g	21	17
Puffed Wheat, breakfast cereal	80	30 g	21	17
Pumpernickel rye kernel bread	50*	30 g	12	6
Pumpkin	75	80 g	4	3
Quik™, chocolate (Nestlé, Australia), dissolved in 1.5% fat milk	41	250 ml	11	5

* Average

FOOD	GI	NOMINAL SERVE SIZE	AVAILABLE CARB PER SERVE	GL PER SERVE
Quik™, strawberry (Nestlé, Australia), dissolved in 1.5% fat milk	35	250 ml	12	4
Raisins	64	60 g	44	28
Ravioli, durum wheat flour, meat filled, boiled	39	180 g	38	15
Real Fruit Bars, strawberry processed fruit bars	90	30 g	26	23
Rice				
Arborio, risotto rice, boiled	69	150 g	43	29
Basmati, boiled	58	150 g	38	22
Calrose brown	87	150 g	40	35
Calrose, white, medium grain, boiled	83	150 g	42	35
Doongara, brown	66	150 g	37	24
Doongara, white	56	150 g	39	22
Instant Doongara, white	94	150 g	42	35
Instant rice, white	87	150 g	42	36
Jasmine rice, white, long-grain	109	150 g	42	46
Long grain, boiled	56	150 g	41	23
Parboiled, Doongara	50	150 g	39	19
Parboiled, Sungold	87	150 g	39	34
Pelde brown	76	150 g	38	29
Pelde, white	93	150 g	43	40
Rice, brown	55	150 g	33	18
Sunbrown Quick™	80	150 g	38	31
Sungold, Pelde, parboiled	87	150 g	43	37
Rice and maize pasta, Ris'O'Mais, gluten-free	76	180 g	49	37
Rice Bran, extruded	19	30 g	14	3
Rice Bubbles™, breakfast cereal	87	30 g	26	22

* Average

FOOD	GI	NOMINAL SERVE SIZE	AVAILABLE CARB PER SERVE	GL PER SERVE
Rice Bubble Treat™ bar	63	30 g	24	15
Rice cakes, white	82	25 g	21	17
Rice Krispies™, breakfast cereal	82	30 g	26	22
Rice noodles, freshly made, boiled	40	180 g	39	15
Rice pasta, brown, boiled 16 min	92	180 g	38	35
Rice vermicelli, dried, boiled	58	180 g	39	22
Rich Tea, 2 biscuits	55	25 g	19	10
Risotto rice, arborio, boiled	69	150 g	43	29
Rockmelon/cantaloupe, raw	65	120 g	6	4
Roggenbrot, Vogel's	59	30 g	14	8
Roll (bread), Kaiser	73	30 g	16	12
Roll-Ups®, processed fruit snack	99	30 g	25	24
Romano beans	46	150 g	18	8
Rye bread, wholemeal	58*	30 g	14	8
Ryvita™ crackers	69	25 g	16	11
Salami	[0]	120 g	0	0
Salmon	0	150 g	0	0
Sao™, plain square crackers	70	25 g	17	12
Sausages, fried	28	100 g	3	1
Scones, plain, made from packet mix	92	25 g	9	8
Sebago potato, peeled, boiled 35 min	87	150 g	17	14
Semolina cooked	55*	150 g	11	6
Shellfish (prawns, crab, lobster etc)	[0]	120 g	0	0
Shortbread biscuits	64	25 g	16	10
Shredded Wheat, breakfast cereal	75*	30 g	20	15
Shredded Wheatmeal™ biscuits	62	25 g	18	11
Skittles®	70	50 g	45	32
Snack foods				
Apricot filled fruit bar	50	50 g	34	17
Burger Rings™	90	50 g	31	28
Chocolate, milk, plain	43	50 g	28	12

* Average

FOOD	GI	NOMINAL SERVE SIZE	AVAILABLE CARB PER SERVE	GL PER SERVE
Chocolate, white, Milky Bar®	44	50 g	29	13
Corn chips, plain, salted	42	50 g	25	11
Heinz Kidz™ Fruit Fingers, banana	61	30 g	20	12
Fruity Bitz™	39	15 g	12	4
Jelly beans	78	30 g	28	22
Life Savers®, peppermint	70	30 g	30	21
M & M's®, peanut	33	30 g	17	6
Mars Bar®	62	60 g	40	25
Muesli bar with dried fruit	61	30 g	21	13
Nutella®	33	20 g	12	4
Popcorn, cooked in microwave	72	20 g	11	8
Pop Tarts™, chocolate	70	50 g	35	24
Potato crisps, plain, salted	57	50 g	18	10
Pretzels	83	30 g	20	16
Real Fruit Bars, strawberry	90	30 g	26	23
Roll-Ups®	99	30 g	25	24
Skittles®	70	50 g	45	32
Snickers Bar®	41	60 g	36	15
Twisties™, cheese flavoured	74	50 g	29	22
Twix®	44	60 g	39	17
So Natural™ soy milk, full-fat (3%), 120 mg calcium, Calciforte	36	250 ml	18	6
So Natural™ soy milk, reduced-fat (1.5%), 120 mg calcium, Light	44	250 ml	17	8
So Natural™ soy milk, full-fat (3%), 0 mg calcium, Original	44	250 ml	17	8
So Natural™ soy smoothie drink, banana, 1% fat	30	250 ml	22	7
So Natural™ soy smoothie drink, chocolate hazelnut, 1% fat	34	250 ml	25	8

* Average

FOOD	GI	NOMINAL SERVE SIZE	AVAILABLE CARB PER SERVE	GL PER SERVE
So Natural™ soy yoghurt, peach and mango, 2% fat, sugar	50	200 ml	26	13
Soft drinks				
Coca Cola®, soft drink	53	250 ml	26	14
Cordial, orange	66	250 ml	20	13
Fanta®, orange soft drink	68	250 ml	34	23
Lucozade®, original	95	250 ml	42	40
Solo™, lemon squash, soft drink	58	250 ml	29	17
Soups				
Black Bean	64	250 ml	27	17
Green Pea, canned	66	250 ml	41	27
Lentil, canned	44	250 ml	21	9
Minestrone, Country Ladle™	39	250 ml	18	7
Split Pea	60	250 ml	27	16
Tomato soup	38	250 ml	17	6
Sourdough rye	48	30 g	12	6
Sourdough wheat	54	30 g	14	8
Soy milk, So Natural™ full-fat (3%), 120 mg calcium, Calciforte	36	250 ml	18	6
Soy milk, So Natural™ reduced-fat (1.5%), 120 mg calcium, Light	44	250 ml	17	8
Soy milk, So Natural™ full-fat (3%), 0 mg calcium, Original	44	250 ml	17	8
Soy smoothie drink, So Natural™ banana, 1% fat	30	250 ml	22	7
Soy smoothie drink, So Natural™ chocolate hazelnut, 1% fat	34	250 ml	25	8
Soy yoghurt, So Natural™ peach and mango, 2% fat, sugar	50	200 g	26	13
Soy beans, dried, boiled	18*	150 g	6	1
Soy beans, canned	14	150 g	6	1

* Average

FOOD	GI	NOMINAL SERVE SIZE	AVAILABLE CARB PER SERVE	GL PER SERVE
Soy-Lin, Bürgen® kibbled soy (8%) and linseed (8%) bread	36	30 g	9	3
Spaghetti, gluten-free, rice and split pea, canned in tomato sauce	68	220 g	27	19
Spaghetti, white, boiled 5 minutes	38*	180 g	48	18
Spaghetti, wholemeal, boiled 5 minutes	37	180 g	42	16
Special K™, breakfast cereal	54	30 g	21	11
Spirali pasta, durum wheat, white, boiled to al denté texture	43	180 g	44	19
Split pea and soy pasta shells, gluten-free	29	180 g	31	9
Split Pea soup	60	250 ml	27	16
Split peas, yellow, boiled 20 min	32	150 g	19	6
Sponge cake, plain	46	63 g	36	17
Sports drinks				
Gatorade®	78	250 ml	15	12
Isostar®	70	250 ml	18	13
Sports Plus®	74	250 ml	17	13
Sustagen Sport®	43	250 ml	49	21
Sports Plus®, sport drink	74	250 ml	17	13
Stoned Wheat Thins crackers	67	25 g	17	12
Strawberries, fresh	40	120 g	3	1
Strawberry jam, regular	51	30 g	20	10
Stuffing, bread	74	30 g	21	16
Sucrose	68*	10 g	10	7
Sugars and honey				
Fructose	19*	10 g	10	2
Glucose	100	10 g	10	10
Iron Bark honey	48	25 g	15	7
Lactose	46*	10 g	10	5
Maltose	105	10 g	10	11

* Average

FOOD	GI	NOMINAL SERVE SIZE	AVAILABLE CARB PER SERVE	GL PER SERVE
Pure Capilano™ honey	58	25 g	21	12
Red Gum honey	46	25 g	18	8
Salvation Jane honey	64	25 g	15	10
Stringy Bark honey	44	25 g	21	9
Sucrose	68*	10 g	10	7
Yapunya honey	52	25 g	17	9
Yellow box honey	35	25 g	18	6
Sultana Bran™, breakfast cereal	73	30 g	19	14
Sultanas	56	60 g	45	25
Sunbrown Quick™ rice, boiled	80	150 g	38	31
Sunflower and barley bread, (Riga)	57	30 g	11	6
Super Supreme pizza, pan (11.4% fat)	36	100 g	24	9
Super Supreme pizza, thin and crispy (13.2% fat)	30	100 g	22	7
Sushi, salmon	48	100 g	36	17
Sustagen™ Hospital with extra fibre, drink made from powdered mix	33	250 ml	44	15
Sustagen™ drink, Dutch Chocolate	31	250 ml	41	13
Sustagen™ pudding, instant vanilla, made from powdered mix	27	250 ml	47	13
Sustagen Sport®, milk-based drink	43	250 ml	49	21
Sustain™, breakfast cereal	68	30 g	22	15
Sustain™ cereal bar	57	30 g	25	14
Swede, cooked	72	150 g	10	7
Sweet corn, whole kernel, canned, drained	46	80 g	14	7
Sweet corn on the cob, boiled	48	80 g	16	8
Sweet potato, cooked	44	150 g	25	11
Sweetened condensed whole milk	61	50 g	28	17
Taco shells, cornmeal-based, baked	68	20 g	12	8
Tapioca, boiled with milk	81	250 ml	18	14

* Average

FOOD	GI	NOMINAL SERVE SIZE	AVAILABLE CARB PER SERVE	GL PER SERVE
Tomato soup	38	250 ml	17	6
Tortellini, cheese, cooked	50	180 g	21	10
TRIM™ custard, reduced-fat	37	100 g	15	6
Tuna	[0]	120 g	0	0
Twisties™, cheese-flavoured, extruded snack, rice and corn	74	50 g	29	22
Twix® Bar, caramel	44	60 g	39	17
Ultra chocolate ice-cream, premium 15% fat (Sara Lee)	37	50 g	9	4
Vaalia™, reduced-fat apricot and mango yoghurt	26	200 g	30	8
Vaalia™, reduced-fat French vanilla yoghurt	26	200 g	10	3
Yoghurt, no-fat, French vanilla, Vaalia, with sugar	40	150 ml	27	10
Yoghurt, no-fat, Mango, Vaalia, with sugar	39	150 ml	25	10
Yoghurt, no-fat, Wildberry, Vaalia, with sugar	38	150 ml	22	8
Yoghurt, no-fat, Strawberry, Vaalia, with sugar	38	150 ml	22	8
Vaalia™, reduced-fat tropical passionfruit yoghurt drink	38	200 ml	29	11
Vanilla cake made from packet mix with vanilla frosting	42	111 g	58	24
Vanilla pudding, instant, made from packet mix and whole milk	40	100 g	16	6
Vanilla wafers, 6 biscuits	77	25 g	18	14
Veal	[0]	120 g	0	0
Vegetables				
Artichokes	[0]	80 g	0	0
Avocado	[0]	80 g	0	0

* Average

FOOD	GI	NOMINAL SERVE SIZE	AVAILABLE CARB PER SERVE	GL PER SERVE
Beetroot	64	80 g	7	5
Bokchoy	[0]	80 g	0	0
Broad beans	79	80 g	11	9
Broccoli	[0]	80 g	0	0
Cabbage	[0]	80 g	0	0
Carrots, peeled, boiled	41*	80 g	5	2
Capsicum	[0]	80 g	0	0
Cauliflower	[0]	80 g	0	0
Celery	[0]	80 g	0	0
Corn on the cob, sweet, boiled	48	80 g	16	8
Cucumber	[0]	80 g	0	0
French beans (runner beans)	[0]	80 g	0	0
Green peas	48	80 g	7	3
Leafy vegetables (spinach, rocket etc)	[0]	80 g	0	0
Lettuce	[0]	80 g	0	0
Parsnips, boiled	97	80 g	12	12
Vermicelli, white, boiled	35	180 g	44	16
Vita-Brits™, breakfast cereal	68	30 g	20	13
Vitari, wild berry, non-dairy, frozen fruit dessert	59	100 g	21	12
Vogel's Honey & Oats bread	55	30 g	14	7
Waffles	76	35 g	13	10
Water crackers	78	25 g	18	14
Watermelon, raw	72	120 g	6	4
Weis Mango Frutia™, low fat frozen fruit dessert	42	100 g	23	10
Weet-Bix™, breakfast cereal	69	30 g	17	12
Wheat-bites™, breakfast cereal	72	30 g	25	18
White bread, wheat flour	70	30 g	14	10
Wholemeal bread, wheat flour	71*	30 g	12	9

* Average

FOOD	GI	NOMINAL SERVE SIZE	AVAILABLE CARB PER SERVE	GL PER SERVE
Wholemeal, sandwich bread (Tip Top)	70	59 g	24	17
Wild About Fruit Apple Juice, pure, clear, unsweetened	44	250 ml	30	13
Wild About Fruit Apple Juice, pure, cloudy, unsweetened	37	250 ml	28	10
Wild About Fruit Apple and mandarin juice	53	250 ml	29	15
Wild About Fruit Apple and mango juice	44	250 ml	27	12
Wonderwhite™ bread	80	30 g	14	11
Yam, peeled, boiled	37*	150 g	36	13
Yoghurt, diet, low fat, no added sugar, vanilla	23	200 ml	13	3
Yoghurt, diet, low fat, no added sugar, (fruit)	24*	200 ml	13	3
Yoghurt drink, Vaalia™, reduced-fat tropical passionfruit	38	200 ml	29	11
Yoghurt, low fat, fruit with artificial sweetener	14	200 ml	13	2
Yoghurt, low fat, fruit with sugar	33	200 ml	31	10
Yoghurt, low fat (0.9%), wild strawberry	31	200 ml	30	9
Yoghurt, no-fat, French vanilla, Vaalia, with sugar	40	150 ml	27	10
Yoghurt, no-fat, Mango, Vaalia, with sugar	39	150 ml	25	10
Yoghurt, no-fat, Wildberry, Vaalia, with sugar	38	150 ml	22	8
Yoghurt, no-fat, Strawberry, Vaalia, with sugar	38	150 ml	22	8

* Average

FOOD CATEGORY
GI VALUES

Many of our readers have asked for GI values to be listed in food categories rather than in A to Z format, for easier access. The categories include: bakery products; beverages; breads; breakfast cereals and bars; cereal grains; cookies; crackers; dairy products; fruit and fruit products; infant formulas; legumes and nuts; meal replacement products; mixed meals and convenience foods; nutritional support products; pasta and noodles; protein foods; snack foods and confectionary; sports bars; soups; sugars; and vegetables.

Within food categories, we have grouped the foods in alphabetical order to help you choose the low GI versions within each category ('this for that') and also to mix and match. If your favourite food has a high GI, check out its glycaemic load. If that's relatively low compared with other foods in that group, then you don't have to worry unduly about its high GI. If it's both high GI and high GL try to cut down the serving size or team it with a very low GI food (e.g. rice (high GI) and lentils (low GI)).

In this food category listing, we have included all the data available, not just average figures and not just Australian data. Here you will find GI values from all over the world, including the United States, Canada, New Zealand, Italy, Sweden, Japan and China among others. Unfortunately there is very little information about the GI of foods used in the UK and Ireland.

As with the A to Z listing we have also included foods that have very little carbohydrate and were omitted from previous editions. However, since so many people ask us for the GI of these foods, we decided to include them and show their GI as [0].

Note: NS means that a brand was not specified.

FOOD	GI	NOMINAL SERVE SIZE	AVAILABLE CARB PER SERVE	GL PER SERVE

BAKERY PRODUCTS

Cakes

FOOD	GI	NOMINAL SERVE SIZE	AVAILABLE CARB PER SERVE	GL PER SERVE
Angel food cake (Loblaw's, Toronto, Canada)	67	50 g	29	19
Banana cake, home made with sugar	47	80 g	38	18
Banana cake, home made without sugar	55	80 g	29	16
Chocolate cake, made from packet mix with chocolate frosting (Betty Crocker)	38	111 g	52	20
Crumpet	69	50 g	19	13
Cupcake, strawberry-iced	73	38 g	26	19
Doughnut, cake type	76	47 g	23	17
Flan cake	65	70 g	48	31
Lamingtons (sponge dipped in chocolate and coconut)	87	50 g	29	25
Pancakes, prepared from shake mix	67	70 g	23	15
Pancakes, buckwheat, gluten-free, made from packet mix (Orgran)	102	77 g	22	22
Pikelets, Golden brand (Tip Top)	85	40 g	21	18
Pound cake (Sara Lee)	54	53 g	28	15
Scones, plain, made from packet mix	92	25 g	9	8
Sponge cake, plain	46	63 g	36	17
Vanilla cake, made from packet mix with vanilla frosting (Betty Crocker)	42	111 g	58	24
Waffles, Aunt Jemima	76	35 g	13	10

Muffins

FOOD	GI	NOMINAL SERVE SIZE	AVAILABLE CARB PER SERVE	GL PER SERVE
Apple, made with sugar	44	60 g	29	13
Apple, made without sugar	48	60 g	19	9

* Average

FOOD	GI	NOMINAL SERVE SIZE	AVAILABLE CARB PER SERVE	GL PER SERVE
Apple, oat, sultana, made from packet mix	54	50 g	26	14
Apricot, coconut and honey, made from packet mix	60	50 g	26	16
Banana, oat and honey, made from packet mix	65	50 g	26	17
Blueberry muffin	59	57 g	29	17
Bran	60	57 g	24	15
Carrot muffin	62	57 g	32	20
Chocolate butterscotch, made from packet mix	53	50 g	28	15
Oatmeal, muffin, made from mix (Quaker Oats)	69	50 g	35	24
Pastry				
Croissant	67	57 g	26	17
Pastry	59	57 g	26	15

BEVERAGES

Alcoholic beverages				
Beer	[0]	250 ml	10	0
Brandy	[0]	30 ml	0	0
Gin	[0]	30 ml	0	0
Red wine	[0]	100 ml	0	0
Sherry	[0]	60 ml	0	0
Whisky	[0]	30 ml	0	0
White wine	[0]	100 ml	0	0
Juices				
Apple juice, pure, unsweetened, (Bern) (Australia)	39			
Apple juice, unsweetened (USA)	40			
Apple juice, unsweetened (Canada)	41			

* Average

FOOD	GI	NOMINAL SERVE SIZE	AVAILABLE CARB PER SERVE	GL PER SERVE
Average of three studies	40	250 ml	29	12
Apple juice, pure, clear, unsweetened (Wild About Fruit, Australia)	44	250 ml	30	13
Apple juice, pure, cloudy, unsweetened (Wild About Fruit, Australia)	37	250 ml	28	10
Carrot juice, freshly made (Sydney, Australia)	43	250 ml	23	10
Cranberry juice cocktail (Ocean Spray®, Australia)	52	250 ml	31	16
Cranberry juice cocktail (Ocean Spray®, USA)	68	250 ml	36	24
Cranberry juice drink (Ocean Spray®, UK)	56	250 ml	29	16
Grapefruit juice, unsweetened (Sunpac, Canada)	48	250 ml	22	11
Orange juice (Canada)	46	250 ml	26	12
Orange juice, unsweetened, (Quelch®, Australia)	53	250 ml	18	9
Pineapple juice, unsweetened (Dole, Canada)	46	250 ml	34	16
Tomato juice, canned, no added sugar (Berri, Australia)	38	250 ml	9	4
Powder drinks				
Build-Up™ with fiber, (Nestlé)	41	250 ml	33	14
Complete Hot Chocolate mix with hot water (Nestlé)	51	250 ml	23	11
Hi-Pro energy drink mix, vanilla, (Harrod)	36	250 ml	19	7
Malted milk in full-fat cow's milk (Nestlé, Australia)	45	250 ml	26	12

* Average

FOOD	GI	NOMINAL SERVE SIZE	AVAILABLE CARB PER SERVE	GL PER SERVE
Milo™ (chocolate nutrient-fortified drink powder)				
Milo™ (Nestlé, Australia), in water	55	250 ml	16	9
Milo™ (Nestlé, Auckland, New Zealand), in water	52	250 ml	16	9
Milo™ (Nestlé, Australia), in full-fat cow's milk	35	250 ml	25	9
Milo™ (Nestlé, New Zealand), in full-fat cow's milk	36	250 ml	26	9
Milo™, (Nestlé, Australia), bottle	30	600 ml	64	19
Milo™, (Nestlé, Australia), tetrapak	35	250 ml	31	11
Nutrimeal™, meal replacement drink, Dutch Chocolate (Usana)	26	250 ml	17	4
Quik™, chocolate (Nestlé, Australia), in water	53	250 ml	7	4
Quik™, chocolate (Nestlé, Australia), in 1.5% fat milk	41	250 ml	11	5
Quik™, strawberry (Nestlé, Australia), in water	64	250 ml	8	5
Quik™, strawberry (Nestlé, Australia), in 1.5% fat milk	35	250 ml	12	4
Smoothies and shakes				
Smoothie, raspberry (Con Agra)	33	250 ml	41	14
Smoothie drink, soy, banana (So Natural)	30	250 ml	22	7
Smoothie drink, soy, chocolate hazelnut (So Natural)	34	250 ml	25	8
Up & Go, cocoa malt flavor (Sanitarium)	43	250 ml	26	11
Up & Go, original malt flavor (Sanitarium)	46	250 ml	24	11

* Average

FOOD	GI	NOMINAL SERVE SIZE	AVAILABLE CARB PER SERVE	GL PER SERVE
Xpress™ chocolate (So Natural, Australia)	39	250 ml	34	13
Yakult® (Yakult, Australia)	46	65 ml	12	6
Soft drinks				
Coca Cola®, soft drink (Australia)	53	250 ml	26	14
Coca Cola®, soft drink/soda (USA)	63	250 ml	26	16
Cordial, orange, reconstituted (Berri)	66	250 ml	20	13
Fanta®, orange soft drink (Australia)	68	250 ml	34	23
Lucozade®, original (sparkling glucose drink)	95	250 ml	42	40
Solo™, lemon squash, soft drink (Australia)	58	250 ml	29	17
Sports drinks				
Gatorade® (Australia)	78	250 ml	15	12
Isostar® (Switzerland)	70	250 ml	18	13
Sports Plus® (Australia)	74	250 ml	17	13
Sustagen Sport® (Australia)	43	250 ml	49	21

BREADS

FOOD	GI	NOMINAL SERVE SIZE	AVAILABLE CARB PER SERVE	GL PER SERVE
Bagel, white, frozen (Canada)	72	70 g	35	25
Baguette, white, plain (France)	95	30 g	15	14
French baguette with chocolate spread (France)	72	70 g	37	27
French baguette with butter and strawberry jam (France)	62	70 g	41	26
Pain au lait (Pasquier, France)	63	60 g	32	20
Bread stuffing, Paxo (Canada)	74	30 g	21	16
Barley flour breads				
100% barley flour (Canada)	67	30 g	13	9
Sunflower and barley bread (Riga, Sydney, Australia)	57	30 g	11	6

* Average

FOOD	GI	NOMINAL SERVE SIZE	AVAILABLE CARB PER SERVE	GL PER SERVE
Fruit Breads				
Fruit and Spice Loaf, thick sliced (Buttercup, Australia)	54	30 g	15	8
Continental fruit loaf, wheat bread with dried fruit (Australia)	47	30 g	15	7
Happiness™ (cinnamon, raisin, pecan bread) (Natural Ovens, USA)	63	30 g	14	9
Muesli bread, made from packet mix in bread oven (Con Agra, USA)	54	30 g	12	7
Gluten-free Bread				
Gluten-free multigrain bread (Country Life Bakeries, Australia)	79	30 g	13	10
Gluten-free white bread, unsliced (gluten-free wheat starch) (UK)	71	30 g	15	11
Gluten-free white bread, sliced (gluten-free wheat starch) (UK)	80	30 g	15	12
mean of two UK studies	76	30 g	15	11
Gluten-free fibre-enriched, unsliced (gluten-free wheat starch, soya bran) (UK)	69	30 g	13	9
Gluten-free fibre-enriched, sliced (gluten-free wheat starch, soya bran) (UK)	76	30 g	13	10
mean of two studies	73	30 g	13	9
Rice Bread				
Rice bread, low-amylose Calrose rice (Pav's, Australia)	72	30 g	12	8
Rice bread, high-amylose Doongara rice (Pav's, Australia)	61	30 g	12	7
Rolls				
Hamburger bun (Loblaw's, Toronto, Canada)	61	30 g	15	9

* Average

FOOD	GI	NOMINAL SERVE SIZE	AVAILABLE CARB PER SERVE	GL PER SERVE
Kaiser rolls (Loblaw's, Canada)	73	30 g	16	12
Rye Bread (pumpernickel)				
Rye kernel bread (Pumpernickel) (Canada)	41	30 g	12	5
Wholegrain pumpernickel (Holtzheuser Brothers Ltd., Toronto, Canada)	46	30 g	11	5
Rye kernel bread, pumpernickel (80% kernels) (Canada)	55	30 g	12	7
Cocktail, sliced (Kasselar Food Products, Toronto, Canada)	55	30 g	12	7
Cocktail, sliced (Kasselar Food Products, Canada)	62	30 g	12	8
Average of six studies	50	30 g	12	6
Wholemeal rye bread	58	30 g	14	8
Specialty rye breads				
Blackbread, Riga (Berzin's, Sydney, Australia)	76	30 g	13	10
Bürgen™ Dark/Swiss rye (Tip Top Bakeries, Australia)	65	30 g	10	7
Klosterbrot wholemeal rye bread (Dimpflmeier, Canada)	67	30 g	13	9
Light rye (Silverstein's, Canada)	68	30 g	14	10
Linseed rye (Rudolph's, Canada)	55	30 g	13	7
Roggenbrot, Vogel's (Stevns & Co, Sydney, Australia)	59	30 g	14	8
Schinkenbrot, Riga (Berzin's, Sydney, Australia)	86	30 g	14	12
Sourdough rye (Canada)	57			
Sourdough rye (Australia)	48			
Average of two studies	53	30 g	12	6

* Average

FOOD	GI	NOMINAL SERVE SIZE	AVAILABLE CARB PER SERVE	GL PER SERVE
Volkornbrot, wholemeal rye bread (Dimpflmeier, Canada)	56	30 g	13	7
Wheat Breads				
Coarse wheat kernel bread, 80% intact kernels (Sweden)	52	30 g	20	10
Spelt wheat breads				
White spelt wheat bread (Slovenia)	74	30 g	23	17
Wholemeal spelt wheat bread (Slovenia)	63	30 g	19	12
Scalded spelt wheat kernel bread (Slovenia)	67	30 g	22	15
Spelt multigrain bread® (Pav's, Australia)	54	30 g	12	7
White wheat flour bread				
White flour (Canada)	69	30 g	14	10
White flour (USA)	70	30 g	14	10
White flour, Sunblest™ (Tip Top, Australia)	70	30 g	14	10
White flour (Dempster's Corporate Foods Ltd., Canada)	71	30 g	14	10
White flour (South Africa)	71	30 g	13	9
White flour (Canada)	71	30 g	14	10
mean of six studies	70	30 g	14	10
White wheat flour bread, hard, toasted (Italian)	73	30 g	15	11
Wonder™, enriched white bread (USA)	73	30 g	14	10
White Turkish bread (Turkey)	87	30 g	17	15
White bread eaten with vinegar as vinaigrette (Sweden)	45	30 g	15	7
White bread eaten with powdered dried seaweed	48	30 g	15	7

* Average

FOOD	GI	NOMINAL SERVE SIZE	AVAILABLE CARB PER SERVE	GL PER SERVE
White bread containing Eurylon® high-amylose maize starch (France)	42	30 g	19	8
White fibre-enriched bread				
White, high-fibre (Dempster's, Canada)	67			
White, high-fibre (Weston's Bakery, Toronto, Canada)	69			
mean of two studies	68	30 g	13	9
White resistant starch-enriched bread				
Fibre White™ (Nature's Fresh, New Zealand)	77	30 g	15	11
Wonderwhite™ (Buttercup, Australia)	80	30 g	14	11
Wholemeal (whole wheat) wheat flour bread				
Wholemeal flour (Canada)	66*	30 g	12	8
Wholemeal flour (USA)	73	30 g	14	10
Wholemeal flour (South Africa)	75	30 g	13	9
Wholemeal flour (Tip Top Bakeries, Australia)	78	30 g	12	9
Wholemeal flour (Kenya)	87	30 g	13	11
Wholemeal Turkish bread	49	30 g	16	8
Specialty wheat breads				
Bürgen® Mixed Grain (Tip Top, Australia)	49*	30 g	11	6
Bürgen® Oat Bran & Honey (Tip Top, Australia)	49	40 g	13	7
Bürgen® Soy-Lin, kibbled soy (8%) and linseed (8%) loaf (Tip Top)	36	30 g	9	3
English Muffin™ bread (Natural Ovens, USA)	77	30 g	14	11

* Average

FOOD	GI	NOMINAL SERVE SIZE	AVAILABLE CARB PER SERVE	GL PER SERVE
Healthy Choice™ Hearty 7 Grain (Con Agra Inc., USA)	55	30 g	14	8
Healthy Choice™ Hearty 100% Whole Grain (Con Agra Inc., USA)	62	30 g	14	9
Helga's™ Classic Seed Loaf (Quality Bakers, Australia)	68	30 g	14	9
Helga's™ traditional wholemeal bread (Quality Bakers, Australia)	70	30 g	13	9
Holsom's wholemeal and rye	63	74 g	28	18
Holsom's sunflower and poppyseed	61	74 g	30	18
Hunger Filler™, whole grain bread (Natural Ovens, USA)	59	30 g	13	7
Molenberg™ (Goodman Fielder, Auckland, New Zealand)	80	30 g	14	11
9 Grain-Multigrain (Tip Top, Australia)	43	30 g	14	6
Nutty Natural™, whole grain bread (Natural Ovens, USA)	59	30 g	12	7
Performax™ (Country Life Bakeries, Australia)	38	30 g	13	5
Ploughman's™ Wholegrain, original recipe (Quality Bakers, Australia)	47	30 g	14	7
Ploughman's™ Wholemeal, smooth milled (Quality Bakers, Australia)	64	30 g	13	9
Semolina Bread (Kenya)	64			
Sourdough wheat (Australia)	54	30 g	14	8
Soy & Linseed bread (packet mix in bread oven) (Con Agra Inc., USA)	50	30 g	10	5
Stay Trim™, whole grain bread (Natural Ovens, USA)	70	30 g	15	10
Sunflower & Barley bread, Riga brand (Berzin's, Australia)	57	30 g	13	7

* Average

FOOD	GI	NOMINAL SERVE SIZE	AVAILABLE CARB PER SERVE	GL PER SERVE
Vogel's Honey & Oats (Stevns & Co., Australia)	55	30 g	14	7
Vogel's Roggenbrot (Stevns & Co., Australia)	59	30 g	14	8
Whole-wheat snack bread (Ryvita Co Ltd., UK)	74	30 g	22	16
100% Whole Grain™ bread (Natural Ovens, USA)	51	30 g	13	7
Unleavened Breads				
Lebanese bread, white (Seda Bakery, Australia)	75	30 g	16	12
Middle Eastern flatbread	97	30 g	16	15
Pita bread, white (Canada)	57	30 g	17	10
Wheat flour flatbread (India)	66	30 g	16	10
Amaranth : wheat (25:75) composite flour flatbread (India)	66	30 g	15	10
Amaranth : wheat (50:50) composite flour flatbread (India)	76	30 g	15	11

BREAKFAST CEREALS AND RELATED PRODUCTS

FOOD	GI	NOMINAL SERVE SIZE	AVAILABLE CARB PER SERVE	GL PER SERVE
All-Bran™ (Kellogg's, Australia)	30	30 g	15	4
All-Bran™ (Kellogg's, USA)	38	30 g	23	9
All-Bran™ (Kellogg's Inc., Canada)	51	30 g	23	9
Average of three studies	40	30 g	21	8
All-Bran Fruit 'n' Oats™ (Kellogg's, Australia)	39	30 g	17	7
All-Bran Soy 'n' Fibre™ (Kellogg's, Australia)	33	30 g	14	4
Amaranth, popped, with milk (India)	97	30 g	19	18
Bran Buds™ (Kellogg's, Canada)	58	30 g	12	7

* Average

FOOD	GI	NOMINAL SERVE SIZE	AVAILABLE CARB PER SERVE	GL PER SERVE
Bran Buds with psyllium (Kellogg's, Canada)	47	30 g	12	6
Bran Chex™ (Nabisco, Canada)	58	30 g	19	11
Bran Flakes™ (Kellogg's, Australia)	74	30 g	18	13
Cheerios™ (General Mills, Canada)	74	30 g	20	15
Chocapic™ (Nestlé, France)	84	30 g	25	21
Coco Pops™ (Kellogg's, Australia)	77	30 g	26	20
Corn Bran™ (Quaker Oats, Canada)	75	30 g	20	15
Corn Chex™ (Nabisco, Canada)	83	30 g	25	21
Cornflakes™ (Kellogg's, New Zealand)	72	30 g	25	18
Cornflakes™ (Kellogg's, Australia)	77	30 g	25	20
Cornflakes™ (Kellogg's, Canada)	83*	30 g	26	22
Cornflakes™ (Kellogg's, USA)	92	30 g	26	24
Average of four studies	81	30 g	26	21
Cornflakes, high-fibre (Presidents Choice, Canada)	74	30 g	23	17
Cornflakes, Crunchy Nut™ (Kellogg's, Australia)	72	30 g	24	17
Corn Pops™ (Kellogg's, Australia)	80	30 g	26	21
Cream of Wheat™ (Nabisco, Canada)	66	250 g	26	17
Cream of Wheat™, Instant (Nabisco, Canada)	74	250 g	30	22
Crispix™ (Kellogg's, Canada)	87	30 g	25	22
Energy Mix™ (Quaker, France)	80	30 g	24	19
Froot Loops™ (Kellogg's, Australia)	69	30 g	26	18
Frosties™, sugar-coated cornflakes (Kellogg's, Australia)	55	30 g	26	15
Fruitful Lite™ (Hubbards, New Zealand)	61	30 g	20	12

* Average

FOOD	GI	NOMINAL SERVE SIZE	AVAILABLE CARB PER SERVE	GL PER SERVE
Fruity-Bix™, berry (Sanitarium, New Zealand)	113	30 g	22	25
Golden Grahams™ (General Mills, Canada)	71	30 g	25	18
Golden Wheats™ (Kellogg's, Australia)	71	30 g	23	16
Grapenuts™ (Post, Kraft, Canada)	67	30 g	19	13
Grapenuts™ (Kraft, USA)	75	30 g	22	16
Average of two studies	71	30 g	21	15
Grapenuts™ Flakes (Post, Canada)	80	30 g	22	17
Guardian™ (Kellogg's, Australia)	37	30 g	12	5
Healthwise™ for bowel health (Uncle Toby's, Australia)	66	30 g	18	12
Healthwise™ for heart health (Uncle Toby's, Australia)	48	30 g	19	9
Honey Rice Bubbles™ (Kellogg's, Australia)	77	30 g	27	20
Honey Smacks™ (Kellogg's, Australia)	71	30 g	23	16
Hot cereal, apple & cinnamon (Con Agra Inc., USA)	37	30 g	22	8
Hot cereal, unflavoured (Con Agra Inc., USA)	25	30 g	19	5
Just Right™ (Kellogg's, Australia)	60	30 g	22	13
Just Right Just Grains™ (Kellogg's, Australia)	62	30 g	23	14
Komplete™ (Kellogg's, Australia)	48	30 g	21	10
Life™ (Quaker Oats Co., Canada)	66	30 g	25	16
Mini Wheats™, whole wheat (Kellogg's, Australia)	58	30 g	21	12
Mini Wheats™, blackcurrant (Kellogg's, Australia)	72	30 g	21	15

* Average

FOOD	GI	NOMINAL SERVE SIZE	AVAILABLE CARB PER SERVE	GL PER SERVE
Muesli (Canada)	66	30 g	24	16
Alpen Muesli (Wheetabix, France)	55	30 g	19	10
Muesli, gluten-free (Freedom Foods, Australia)	39	30 g	19	7
Muesli, Lite (Sanitarium, New Zealand)	54	30 g	18	10
Muesli, Natural (Sanitarium, New Zealand)	57	30 g	19	11
Muesli, Natural (Sanitarium, Australia)	40	30 g	19	8
Muesli, No Name (Sunfresh, Canada)	60	30 g	18	11
Muesli, Swiss Formula (Uncle Toby's, Australia)	56	30 g	16	9
Muesli, toasted (Purina, Australia)	43	30 g	17	7
Nutrigrain™ (Kellogg's, Australia)	66	30 g	15	10
Oat 'n' Honey Bake™ (Kellogg's, Australia)	77	30 g	17	13
Oat bran, raw (Quaker Oats, Canada)	50	10 g	5	2
Oat bran, raw	59	10 g	5	3
Average of two studies	55	10 g	5	3
Porridge (Uncle Toby's, Australia)	42	250 g	21	9
Porridge (Canada)	49	250 g	23	11
Traditional porridge oats (Lowan, Australia)	51	250 g	21	11
Porridge (Hubbards, New Zealand)	58	250 g	21	12
Porridge (Australia)	58	250 g	21	12
Porridge (Canada)	62	250 g	23	14
Porridge (Canada)	69	250 g	23	16
Porridge (USA)	75	250 g	23	17
Average of eight studies	58	250 g	22	13
Quick Oats (Quaker Oats, Canada)	65	250 g	26	17

* Average

FOOD	GI	NOMINAL SERVE SIZE	AVAILABLE CARB PER SERVE	GL PER SERVE
One Minute Oats (Quaker Oats, Canada)	66	250 g	26	17
Average of two studies	66	250 g	26	17
Pop Tarts™, Double Chocolate (Kellogg's, Australia)	70	50 g	36	25
Pro Stars™ (General Mills, Canada)	71	30 g	24	17
Puffed Wheat (Quaker Oats, Canada)	67	30 g	20	13
Puffed Wheat (Sanitarium, Australia)	80	30 g	21	17
Average of two studies	74	30 g	21	16
Raisin Bran™ (Kellogg's, USA)	61	30 g	19	12
Red River Cereal (Maple Leaf Mills, Canada)	49	30 g	22	11
Rice Bran, extruded (Rice Growers, Australia)	19	30 g	14	3
Rice Bubbles™ (Kellogg's, Australia)	87*	30 g	26	22
Rice Chex™ (Nabisco, Canada)	89	30 g	26	23
Rice Krispies™ (Kellogg's, Canada)	82	30 g	26	22
Shredded Wheat (Canada)	67	30 g	20	13
Shredded Wheat™ (Nabisco, Canada)	83	30 g	20	17
Average of two studies	75	30 g	20	15
Special K™ (Kellogg's, Australia)	54	30 g	21	11
Special K™ (Kellogg's, USA)	69	30 g	21	14
Special K™ (Kellogg's, France)	84	30 g	24	20
Soy Tasty™ (Sanitarium, Australia)	60	30 g	20	12
Soytana™ (Vogel's, Australia)	49	45 g	25	12
Sultana Bran™ (Kellogg's, Australia)	73	30 g	19	14
Sustain™ (Kellogg's, Australia)	68	30 g	22	15
Team™ (Nabisco, Canada)	82	30 g	22	17
Thank Goodness™ (Hubbards, New Zealand)	65	30 g	23	15

* Average

FOOD	GI	NOMINAL SERVE SIZE	AVAILABLE CARB PER SERVE	GL PER SERVE
Total™ (General Mills, Canada)	76	30 g	22	17
Ultra-bran™ (Vogel's, Australia)	41	30 g	13	5
Wheat-bites™ (Uncle Toby's, Australia)	72	30 g	25	18
Whole wheat Goldies™ (Kellogg's, Australia)	70	30 g	20	14
Good Start™, muesli wheat biscuits (Sanitarium, Australia)	68	30 g	20	14
Hi-Bran Weet-Bix™, wheat biscuits (Sanitarium, Australia)	61	30 g	17	10
Hi-Bran Weet-Bix™ with soy and linseed (Sanitarium, Australia)	57	30 g	16	9
Honey Goldies™ (Kellogg's Australia)	72	30 g	21	15
Lite-Bix™, plain, no added sugar (Sanitarium, Australia)	70	30 g	20	14
Oat bran Weet-Bix™ (Sanitarium, Australia)	57	30 g	20	11
Sultana Goldies™ (Kellogg's Australia)	65	30 g	21	13

BREAKFAST CEREAL BARS

FOOD	GI	NOMINAL SERVE SIZE	AVAILABLE CARB PER SERVE	GL PER SERVE
Crunchy Nut Cornflakes™ bar (Kellogg's, Australia)	72	30 g	26	19
Fibre Plus™ bar (Uncle Toby's, Australia)	78	30 g	23	18
Fruity-Bix™ bar, fruit and nut (Sanitarium, Australia)	56	30 g	19	10
Fruity-Bix™ bar, wild berry (Sanitarium, Australia)	51	30 g	19	9
K-Time Just Right™ bar (Kellogg's, Australia)	72	30 g	24	17

* Average

FOOD	GI	NOMINAL SERVE SIZE	AVAILABLE CARB PER SERVE	GL PER SERVE
K-Time Strawberry Crunch™ bar (Kellogg's, Australia)	77	30 g	25	19
Rice Bubble Treat™ bar (Kellogg's, Australia)	63	30 g	24	15
Sustain™ bar (Kellogg's, Australia)	57	30 g	25	14

CEREAL GRAINS

FOOD	GI	NOMINAL SERVE SIZE	AVAILABLE CARB PER SERVE	GL PER SERVE
Amaranth popped, with milk	97	30 g	22	21
Barley				
Barley, pearled (Canada)	22			
Barley (Canada)	22			
Barley, pot, boiled 20 min	25			
Barley (Canada)	27			
Barley, pearled (Canada)	29			
Average of five studies	25	150 g	32	8
Barley, cracked (Malthouth, Tunisia)	50	150 g	42	21
Barley, rolled cooked, dry (Australia)	66	50 g	38	25
Buckwheat				
Buckwheat (Canada)	54*	150 g	30	16
Buckwheat groats, boiled 12 min (Sweden)	45	150 g	30	13
Corn/Maize				
Maize (Zea mays), flour made into chapatti (India)	59			
Maize meal porridge/gruel (Kenya)	109			
Cornmeal				
Cornmeal, boiled in salted water 2 min (Canada)	68	150 g	13	9
Cornmeal with margarine (Canada)	69	150 g	12	9
Average of two studies	69	150 g	13	9

* Average

FOOD	GI	NOMINAL SERVE SIZE	AVAILABLE CARB PER SERVE	GL PER SERVE
Corn, sweet				
Corn, sweet, 'Honey & Pearl' variety boiled (New Zealand)	37	150 g	30	11
Corn, sweet, on the cob, boiled 20 min (Australia)	48	150 g	30	14
Corn, sweet, (Canada)	59	150 g	33	20
Corn, sweet, (USA)	60	150 g	33	20
Corn, sweet, (South Africa)	62	150 g	33	20
Average of three studies	53	150 g	32	17
Sweet corn, canned, diet-pack (USA)	46	150 g	28	13
Sweet corn, frozen, reheated in microwave (Canada)	47	150 g	33	16
Taco shells, cornmeal-based, baked (Old El Paso, Canada)	68	20 g	12	8
Couscous				
Couscous, boiled 5 min (USA)	61			
Couscous, boiled 5 min (Tunisia)	69			
Average of two studies	65	150 g	35	23
Millet				
Millet, boiled (Canada)	71	150 g	36	25
Rice, white				
Arborio, risotto rice, boiled (Sun Rice, Australia)	69	150 g	43	29
White (*Oryza sativa*), boiled (India)	69	150 g	43	30
Rice, boiled white				
Type NS (France)	45*	150 g	30	14
Type NS (India)	48	150 g	38	18
Type NS (France)	52	150 g	36	19
Type NS (Pakistan)	69	150 g	38	26

* Average

FOOD	GI	NOMINAL SERVE SIZE	AVAILABLE CARB PER SERVE	GL PER SERVE
Type NS (Canada)	60*	150 g	42	25
Type NS, boiled in salted water (India)	72	150 g	38	27
Type NS, boiled 13 min (Italy)	102	150 g	30	31
Type NS (Kenya)	112	150 g	42	47
Type NS, boiled in salted water, refrigerated 16–20h, reheated (India)	53	150 g	38	20
Type NS, boiled 13 min, then baked 10 min (Italy)	104	150 g	30	31
Rice, Long grain, boiled				
Long grain, boiled 5 min (Canada)	41	150 g	40	16
Long grain, boiled 15 min (Mahatma, Australia)	50	150 g	43	21
Long grain (Uncle Bens®, New Zealand)	56	150 g	43	24
Long grain, boiled 25 min (Surinam)	56	150 g	43	24
Long grain, boiled 15 min	58	150 g	40	23
Gem long grain (Dainty, Canada)	58*	150 g	40	23
Long grain, boiled 7 min (Star, Canada)	64	150 g	40	26
Average of seven studies	55	150 g	41	23
Rice, long grain, quick-cooking varieties				
Long grain, parboiled 10 min cooking time (Uncle Ben's, Belgium)	68	150 g	37	25
Long grain, parboiled, 20 min cooking time (Uncle Ben's, Belgium)	75	150 g	37	28
Long grain, microwaved 2 min (Express Rice, Masterfoods, UK)	52	150 g	37	19

* Average

FOOD	GI	NOMINAL SERVE SIZE	AVAILABLE CARB PER SERVE	GL PER SERVE
Rice, specialty rices				
Cajun Style, Uncle Ben's® (Effem Foods, Canada)	51	150 g	37	19
Garden Style, Uncle Ben's® (Effem Foods, Canada)	55	150 g	37	21
Long Grain and Wild, Uncle Ben's® (Effem Foods, Canada)	54	150 g	37	20
Mexican Fast and Fancy, Uncle Ben's® (Effem Foods, Canada)	58	150 g	37	22
Saskatchewan wild rice (Canada)	57	150 g	32	18
Broken rice, white (Lion Foods, Thailand)	86	150 g	43	37
Glutinous rice, white (Thailand)	98	150 g	32	31
Jasmine rice, white, long grain (Thailand)	109	150 g	42	46
Rice, white low-amylose				
Calrose, white, medium grain, boiled (Rice Growers, Australia)	83	150 g	42	35
Sungold, Pelde, parboiled (Rice Growers, Australia)	87	150 g	43	37
Waxy (0–2% amylose) (Rice Growers, Australia)	88	150 g	43	38
Pelde, white (Rice Growers, Australia)	93	150 g	43	40
White, low-amylose, boiled (Turkey)	139	150 g	43	60
Rice, white high-amylose				
Bangladeshi rice variety BR16 (28% amylose)	37	150 g	39	14
Bangladeshi rice variety BR16, long-grain (27% amylose)	39	150 g	39	15
Average of two studies	38	150 g	39	15

* Average

FOOD	GI	NOMINAL SERVE SIZE	AVAILABLE CARB PER SERVE	GL PER SERVE
Doongara, white (Rice Growers, Australia)	56*	150 g	42	24
Koshikari (Japonica), short-grain, (Japan)	48	150 g	42	20
Rice, Basmati				
Basmati, boiled (Mahatma, Australia)	58	150 g	42	24
Precooked basmati rice, Uncle Ben's Express® (UK)	57	150 g	41	24
Quick-cooking basmati, Uncle Ben's® Superior (Belgium)	60	150 g	38	23
Rice, brown				
Brown (Canada)	66	150 g	33	21
Brown, steamed (USA)	50	150 g	33	16
Brown (Oriza Sativa), boiled (South India)	50	150 g	33	16
Average of three studies	55	150 g	33	18
Calrose brown (Rice Growers, Australia)	87	150 g	40	35
Doongara brown, high-amylose (Rice Growers, Australia)	66	150 g	37	24
Pelde brown (Rice Growers, Australia)	76	150 g	38	29
Parboiled, cooked 20 min, Uncle Ben's Natur-reis ® (Belgium)	64	150 g	36	23
Sunbrown Quick™ (Rice Growers, Australia)	80	150 g	38	31
Rice Instant/puffed				
Instant rice, white, boiled 1 min (Canada)	46	150 g	42	19
Instant rice, white, cooked 6 min (Trice brand, Australia)	87	150 g	42	36

* Average

FOOD	GI	NOMINAL SERVE SIZE	AVAILABLE CARB PER SERVE	GL PER SERVE
Puffed, white, cooked 5 min, Uncle Ben's Snabbris® (Belgium)	74	150 g	42	31
Average of three studies	69	150 g	42	29
Instant Doongara, white, cooked 5 min (Rice Growers, Australia)	94	150 g	42	35
Rice parboiled				
Parboiled rice (Canada)	48	150 g	36	18
Parboiled rice (USA)	72	150 g	36	26
Converted, white, Uncle Ben's® (Canada)	45	150 g	36	16
Converted, white, boiled 20–30 min, Uncle Ben's® (USA)	38	150 g	36	14
Converted, white, long grain, boiled 20–30 min, Uncle Ben's® (USA)	50	150 g	36	18
Boiled, 12 min (Denmark)	43	150 g	36	15
Long grain, boiled 5 min (Canada)	38	150 g	36	14
Long grain, boiled, 10 min (USA)	61	150 g	36	22
Long grain, boiled 15 min (Canada)	47	150 g	36	17
Long grain, boiled 25 min (Canada)	46	150 g	36	17
Average of four studies	49	150 g	36	18
Rice parboiled, low-amylose				
Bangladeshi rice variety BR2, parboiled (12% amylose)	51	150 g	38	19
Parboiled, Sungold (Rice Growers, Australia)	87	150 g	39	34
Rice parboiled, high-amylose				
Parboiled, high-amylose (28%), Doongara (Rice Growers, Australia)	50	150 g	42	21
Bangladeshi rice variety BR16 (28% amylose)	35	150 g	37	13

* Average

FOOD	GI	NOMINAL SERVE SIZE	AVAILABLE CARB PER SERVE	GL PER SERVE
Bangladeshi rice variety BR16, traditional method (27% amylose)	32	150 g	38	12
Bangladeshi rice variety BR16, pressure parboiled (27% amylose)	27	150 g	41	11
Bangladeshi rice variety BR4 (27% amylose)	33	150 g	38	13
Average	35	150 g	39	14
Rye, whole kernels				
Rye, whole kernels, dry (Canada)	29	50 g	38	11
Average of three studies	34	50 g	38	13
Wheat				
Wheat, whole kernels				
Wheat, whole kernels, dry (Triticum aestivum) (India)	30	50 g	38	11
Wheat, whole kernels, dry (Canada)	42	50 g	33	14
Wheat, whole kernels, pressure cooked, dry (Canada)	44	50 g	33	14
Wheat, whole kernels, dry (Canada)	48	50 g	33	16
Average of four studies	41	50 g	34	14
Wheat, type NS, dry (India)	90	50 g	38	34
Wheat, precooked kernels				
Durum wheat, precooked, cooked 20 min, dry (France)	52	50 g	37	19
Durum wheat, precooked, cooked 10 min, dry (France)	50	50 g	33	17
Durum wheat, precooked in pouch, reheated (France)	40	125 g	39	16
Quick-cooking (White Wings, Australia)	54	150 g	47	25

* Average

FOOD	GI	NOMINAL SERVE SIZE	AVAILABLE CARB PER SERVE	GL PER SERVE
Semolina				
Semolina, roasted at 105°C then gelatinised with water (India)	55			
Semolina, steamed and gelatinised (India)	54			
Average of two studies	55	150 g	11	6
Wheat cracked (bulghur)				
Bulghur, boiled	47	150 g	26	12

COOKIES

FOOD	GI	NOMINAL SERVE SIZE	AVAILABLE CARB PER SERVE	GL PER SERVE
Arrowroot (McCormicks's, Canada)	63	25 g	20	13
Arrowroot plus (McCormicks's, Canada)	62	25 g	18	11
Milk Arrowroot™ (Arnotts, Australia)	69	25 g	18	12
Average of three studies	65	25 g	19	12
Barquette Abricot (LU, France)	71	40 g	32	23
Bebe Dobre Rano Chocolate (LU, Czech Republic)	57	50 g	33	19
Bebe Dobre Rano Honey and Hazelnuts (LU, Czech Republic)	51	50 g	34	17
Bebe Jemne Susenky (LU, Czech Republic)	67	25 g	20	14
Digestives	59	25 g	16	10
Digestives, gluten-free (Nutricia, UK)	58	25 g	17	10
Evergreen met Krenten (LU, Netherlands)	66	38 g	21	14
Golden Fruit (Griffin's, New Zealand)	77	25 g	17	13
Graham Wafers (Christie Brown, Canada)	74	25 g	18	14

* Average

FOOD	GI	NOMINAL SERVE SIZE	AVAILABLE CARB PER SERVE	GL PER SERVE
Gran'Dia Banana, Oats and Honey (LU, Brazil)	28	30 g	23	6
Grany en-cas Abricot (LU, France)	55	30 g	16	9
Grany en-cas Fruits des bois (LU, France)	50	30 g	14	7
Grany Rush Apricot (LU, Netherlands)	62	30 g	20	12
Highland Oatmeal™ (Westons, Australia)	55	25 g	18	10
Highland Oatcakes (Walker's, Scotland)	57	25 g	15	8
LU P'tit Déjeuner Chocolat (LU, France)	42	50 g	34	14
LU P'tit Déjeuner Miel et Pépites Chocolat (LU, France)	49*	50 g	35	17
Maltmeal wafer (Griffin's, New Zealand)	50	25 g	17	9
Morning Coffee™ (Arnotts, Australia)	79	25 g	19	15
Nutrigrain Fruits des bois (Kellogg's, France)	57	35 g	23	13
Oatmeal (Canada)	54	25 g	17	9
Oro (Saiwa, Italy)	64*	40 g	32	20
Petit LU Normand (LU, France)	51	25 g	19	10
Petit LU Roussillon (LU, France)	48	25 g	18	9
Prince Energie+ (LU, France)	73	25 g	17	13
Prince fourré chocolat (LU, France)	52*	65 g	30	16
Prince Meganana Chocolate (LU, Spain)	49	50 g	36	18
Prince Petit Déjeuner Vanille (LU, France and Spain)	45	50 g	36	16

* Average

FOOD	GI	NOMINAL SERVE SIZE	AVAILABLE CARB PER SERVE	GL PER SERVE
Rich Tea (Canada)	55	25 g	19	10
Sablé des Flandres (LU, France)	57	20 g	15	8
Shortbread (Arnotts, Australia)	64	25 g	16	10
Shredded Wheatmeal™ (Arnotts, Australia)	62	25 g	18	11
Snack Right Fruit Slice (97% fat-free) (Arnott's, Australia)	48	25 g	19	9
Thé (France)	41	20 g	16	6
Vanilla Wafers (Christie Brown, Canada)	77	25 g	18	14
Véritable Petit Beurre (LU, France)	51	25 g	18	9

CRACKERS

FOOD	GI	NOMINAL SERVE SIZE	AVAILABLE CARB PER SERVE	GL PER SERVE
Breton wheat crackers (Dare Foods, Canada)	67	25 g	14	10
Corn Thins, puffed corn cakes, gluten-free (Real Foods, Australia)	87	25 g	20	18
Cream Cracker (LU, Brazil)	65	25 g	17	11
High-calcium cracker (Danone, Malaysia)	52	25 g	17	9
Jatz™, plain salted cracker biscuits (Arnotts, Australia)	55	25 g	17	10
Puffed Crispbread (Westons, Australia)	81	25 g	19	15
Puffed rice cakes (Rice Growers, Australia)	82	25 g	21	17
Rye crispbread (Canada)	63	25 g	16	10
Ryvita™ (Canada)	69	25 g	16	11
High-fibre rye crispbread (Ryvita, UK)	59	25 g	15	9
Rye crispbread (Ryvita, UK)	63	25 g	18	11

* Average

FOOD	GI	NOMINAL SERVE SIZE	AVAILABLE CARB PER SERVE	GL PER SERVE
Average of four studies	64	25 g	16	11
Kavli™ Norwegian Crispbread (Players, Australia)	71	25 g	16	12
Sao™, plain square crackers (Arnotts, Australia)	70	25 g	17	12
Stoned Wheat Thins (Christie Brown, Canada)	67	25 g	17	12
Water cracker (Canada)	63	25 g	18	11
Water cracker (Arnotts, Australia)	78	25 g	18	14
Average of two studies	71	25 g	18	13
Premium Soda Crackers (Christie Brown, Canada)	74	25 g	17	12
Vita-wheat™, original, crispbread (Arnott's, Australia)	55	25 g	19	10

DAIRY PRODUCTS AND ALTERNATIVES

Custard

No Bake Egg Custard (Nestlé, Australia)	35	100 g	17	6
Custard, home made (Australia)	43	100 g	17	7
TRIM™, reduced-fat custard (Pauls, Australia)	37	100 g	15	6
Average of three studies	38	100 g	16	6

Ice-cream, Regular/NS

Ice-cream, NS (Canada)	36			
Ice-cream (half vanilla, half chocolate) (Italy)	57			
Ice-cream, NS (USA)	62			
Ice-cream, chocolate flavored (USA)	68			
Ice-cream (half vanilla, half chocolate) (Italy)	80			

* Average

FOOD	GI	NOMINAL SERVE SIZE	AVAILABLE CARB PER SERVE	GL PER SERVE
Average of five studies	61	50 g	13	8
Ice-cream, reduced or low fat				
Ice-cream, vanilla, (Peter's, Australia)	50	50 g	6	3
Ice-cream, (1.2 % fat), Prestige Light vanilla (Norco, Australia)	47	50 g	10	5
Ice-cream, (1.4% fat), Prestige Light toffee (Norco, Australia)	37	50 g	14	5
Ice-cream, Prestige Golden macadamia (Norco, Australia)	37	50 g	9	3
Ice-cream, premium				
Ice-cream, Ultra chocolate, 15% fat (Sara Lee, Australia)	37	50 g	9	4
Ice-cream, French vanilla, 16% fat (Sara Lee, Australia)	38	50 g	9	3
Milk				
Full-fat (Italy)	11			
Full-fat (3% fat, Sweden)	21			
Full-fat (Italy)	24			
Full-fat (Australia)	31			
Full-fat (Canada)	34			
Full-fat (USA)	40			
Average of five studies	27	250 ml	12	3
Fermented cow's milk (ropy milk, Sweden)	11			
Fermented cow's milk (filmjölk, Sweden)	11			
Average of two foods	11			
Milk, skim (Canada)	32	250 g	13	4
Milk, condensed, sweetened (Nestlé, Australia)	61	50 g	28	17

* Average

FOOD	GI	NOMINAL SERVE SIZE	AVAILABLE CARB PER SERVE	GL PER SERVE
Milk, low fat, chocolate, with aspartame, Lite White™ (Australia)	24	250 g	15	3
Milk, low fat, chocolate, with sugar, Lite White™ (Australia)	34	250 g	26	9
Mousse, reduced-fat, made from mix with water				
Butterscotch, 1.9% fat (Nestlé, Australia)	36	50 g	10	4
Chocolate, 2% fat (Nestlé, Australia)	31	50 g	11	3
French vanilla, 2% fat (Nestlé, Australia)	42	100 ml	6	3
Hazelnut, 2.4% fat (Nestlé, Australia)	36	50 g	10	4
Mango, 1.8% fat (Nestlé, Australia)	33	50 g	11	4
Mixed berry, 2.2% fat (Nestlé, Australia)	36	50 g	10	4
Strawberry, 2.3% fat (Nestlé, Australia)	32	50 g	10	3
Average of six foods	34	50 g	10	4
Pudding				
Instant, chocolate, made from powder and milk (White Wings, Australia)	47	100 g	16	7
Instant, vanilla, made from powder and milk (White Wings, Australia)	40	100 g	16	6
Average of two foods	44	100 g	16	7
Yoghurt				
Yoghurt, type (Canada)	36	200 g	9	3
Yoghurt low fat				
Low fat, fruit, aspartame, Ski™ (Dairy Farmers, Australia)	14	200 g	13	2

* Average

FOOD	GI	NOMINAL SERVE SIZE	AVAILABLE CARB PER SERVE	GL PER SERVE
Low fat, fruit, sugar, Ski™ (Dairy Farmers, Australia)	33	200 g	31	10
Low fat (0.9%), fruit, wild strawberry (Ski d'lite™, Dairy Farmers, Australia)	31	200 g	30	9
Yoghurt diet non-fat, with low-calorie sweeteners (no added sugars)				
Yoghurt, no-fat, French Vanilla, Vaalia, with sugar	40	150 g	27	10
Yoghurt, no-fat, Mango, Vaalia, with sugar	39	150 g	25	10
Yoghurt, no-fat, Wildberry, Vaalia, with sugar	38	150 g	22	8
Yoghurt, no-fat, Strawberry, Vaalia, with sugar	38	150 g	22	8
Diet Vaalia™, vanilla (Pauls, Australia)	23	200 g	13	3
mean of five foods	24	200 g	14	3
Yoghurt reduced-fat				
Reduced-fat, Vaalia™, apricot & mango (Pauls, Australia)	26	200 g	30	8
Reduced-fat, Vaalia™, French vanilla (Pauls, Australia)	26	200 g	10	3
Reduced-fat, Extra-Lite™, strawberry (Pauls, Australia)	28	200 g	33	9
mean of three foods	27	200 g	24	7
Yoghurt drink, reduced-fat, Vaalia™, passionfruit (Pauls, Australia)	38	200 g	29	11
Soy-based dairy product alternatives				
Soy milks (containing maltodextrin)				
Soy milk, full-fat, Original (So Natural, Australia)	44	250 g	17	8

* Average

FOOD	GI	NOMINAL SERVE SIZE	AVAILABLE CARB PER SERVE	GL PER SERVE
Soy milk, full-fat, Calciforte (So Natural, Australia)	36	250 g	18	6
Soy milk, reduced-fat, Light (So Natural, Australia)	44	250 g	17	8
Soy milk drinks				
Soy smoothie drink, banana, 1% fat (So Natural, Australia)	30	250 g	22	7
Soy smoothie drink, chocolate hazelnut, 1% fat (So Natural, Australia)	34	250 g	25	8
mean of two drinks	32	250 g	23	7
Up & Go™, cocoa malt flavour (Sanitarium, Australia)	43	250 g	26	11
Up & Go™, original malt flavour (Sanitarium, Australia)	46	250 g	24	11
Average of two drinks	45	250 g	25	11
Xpress™, chocolate (So Natural, Australia)	39	250 g	34	13
Soy yoghurt				
Soy yoghurt, peach and mango, 2% fat, sugar (So Natural, Australia)	50	200 g	26	13
Tofu-based frozen dessert, chocolate (USA)	115	50 g	9	10

FRUIT AND FRUIT PRODUCTS

FOOD	GI	NOMINAL SERVE SIZE	AVAILABLE CARB PER SERVE	GL PER SERVE
Apple, (Denmark)	28	120 g	13	4
Apple, Braeburn (New Zealand)	32	120 g	13	4
Apple, s (Canada)	34	120 g	16	5
Apple, Golden Delicious (Canada)	39	120 g	16	6
Apple, (USA)	40	120 g	16	6

* Average

FOOD	GI	NOMINAL SERVE SIZE	AVAILABLE CARB PER SERVE	GL PER SERVE
Apple, (Italy)	44	120 g	13	6
Average of six studies	38	120 g	15	6
Apple, dried (Australia)	29	60 g	34	10
Apple juice, unsweetened, reconstituted (Berri, Australia)	39	250 g	25	10
Apple juice, unsweetened (USA)	40	250 g	29	12
Apple juice, unsweetened (Allens, Canada)	41	250 g	30	12
Average of three studies	40	250 g	28	11
Apricots, raw (Italy)	57	120 g	9	5
Apricots, canned in light syrup (Riviera, Canada)	64	120 g	19	12
Apricots, dried (Australia)	30	60 g	27	8
Apricots, dried (Wasco, Canada)	32	60 g	30	10
Average of two studies	31	60 g	28	9
Apricot fruit bar, (Mother Earth, New Zealand)	50	50 g	34	17
Apricot fruit spread, (Glen Ewin, Australia)	55	30 g	13	7
Apricot Fruity Bitz™ (Blackmores, Australia)	42	15 g	12	5
Banana (Canada)	46	120 g	25	12
Banana (Italy)	58	120 g	23	13
Banana (Canada)	58	120 g	25	15
Banana (Canada)	62	120 g	25	16
Banana (South Africa)	70	120 g	23	16
Banana, ripe (all yellow) (USA)	51	120 g	25	13
Banana, under-ripe (Denmark)	30	120 g	21	6
Banana, slightly under-ripe (yellow with green sections) (USA)	42	120 g	25	11

* Average

FOOD	GI	NOMINAL SERVE SIZE	AVAILABLE CARB PER SERVE	GL PER SERVE
Banana, over-ripe (yellow flecked with brown) (USA)	48	120 g	25	12
Banana, over-ripe (Denmark)	52	120 g	20	11
Average of 10 studies	52	120 g	24	12
Banana, processed fruit fingers, Heinz Kidz™ (Australia)	61	30 g	20	12
Breadfruit (Artocarpus altilis), raw (Australia)	68	120 g	27	18
Cherries, raw, NS[8] (Canada)	22	120 g	12	3
Chico (Zapota zapotilla coville), raw (Philippines)	40	120 g	29	12
Cranberry juice cocktail (Ocean Spray, Australia)	52	250 g	31	16
Cranberry juice cocktail (Ocean Spray, USA)	68	250 g	35	24
Cranberry juice drink (Ocean Spray®, UK)	56	250 g	29	16
Custard apple, raw, flesh only (Australia)	54	120 g	19	10
Dates, dried (Australia)	103	60 g	40	42
Figs, dried, tenderised (Dessert Maid, Australia)	61	60 g	26	16
Fruit Cocktail, canned (Delmonte, Canada)	55	120 g	16	9
Grapefruit, raw (Canada)	25	120 g	11	3
Grapefruit juice, unsweetened (Sunpac, Canada)	48	250 g	20	9
Grapes, NS (Canada)	43	120 g	17	7
Grapes, NS (Italy)	49	120 g	19	9
Average of two studies	46	120 g	18	8
Grapes, black, Waltham Cross (Australia)	59	120 g	18	11

* Average

FOOD	GI	NOMINAL SERVE SIZE	AVAILABLE CARB PER SERVE	GL PER SERVE
Kiwi fruit, Hayward (New Zealand)	47	120 g	12	5
Kiwi fruit (Australia)	58	120 g	12	7
Average of two studies	53	120 g	12	6
Lychee, canned in syrup and drained, Narcissus brand (China)	79	120 g	20	16
Mango (*Mangifera indica*) (Philippines)	41	120 g	20	8
Mango (Mangifera indica) (Australia)	51	120 g	15	8
Mango, ripe (*Mangifera indica*) (India)	60	120 g	15	9
Average of three studies	51	120 g	17	8
Mango, Frutia™ (Weis, Australia)	42	100 g	23	10
Marmalade, orange (Australia)	48	30 g	20	9
Oranges, NS (Denmark)	31	120 g	11	3
Oranges, NS (South Africa)	33	120 g	10	3
Oranges, NS (Canada)	40	120 g	11	4
Oranges, NS s (Italy)	48	120 g	11	5
Oranges (Sunkist, USA)	48	120 g	11	5
Oranges NS (Canada)	51	120 g	11	6
Average of six studies	42	120 g	11	5
Orange juice (Canada)	46	250 g	26	12
Orange juice, reconstituted (Quelch, Australia)	53	250 g	18	9
Orange juice, reconstituted from frozen concentrate (USA)	57	250 g	26	15
Average of three studies	52	250 g	23	12
Paw paw (Carica papaya) (Australia)	56	120 g	8	5
Paw paw, ripe (India)	60	120 g	29	17
Papaya (*Carica papaya*) (Philippines)	60	120 g	15	9
Average of three studies	59	120 g	17	10
Peach, raw (Canada)	28	120 g	13	4
Peach, raw (Italy)	56	120 g	8	5
Average of two studies	42	120 g	11	5

* Average

FOOD	GI	NOMINAL SERVE SIZE	AVAILABLE CARB PER SERVE	GL PER SERVE
Peach, canned in natural juice (Ardmona, Australia)	30	120 g	11	3
Peach, canned in natural juice (SPC, Australia)	45	120 g	11	5
Average of two studies	38	120 g	11	4
Peach, canned in heavy syrup (Letona, Australia)	58	120 g	15	9
Peach, canned in light syrup (Delmonte, Canada)	52	120 g	18	9
Peach, canned in reduced-sugar syrup (SPC, Australia)	62	120 g	17	11
Pear, raw, NS (Canada)	33	120 g	13	4
Pear, Winter Nellis, raw (New Zealand)	34	120 g	12	4
Pear, Bartlett, raw (Canada)	41	120 g	8	3
Pear, raw NS (Italy)	42	120 g	11	4
Average of four studies	38	120 g	11	4
Pear halves, canned in reduced-sugar syrup, SPC Lite (Australia)	25	120 g	14	4
Pear halves, canned in natural juice (SPC, Australia)	43	120 g	13	5
Pear, canned in pear juice, Bartlett (Delmonte, Canada)	44	120 g	11	5
Pineapple, raw (Australia)	66	120 g	10	6
Pineapple (*Ananas comosus*), raw (Philippines)	51	120 g	16	8
Average of two studies	59	120 g	13	7
Pineapple juice, unsweetened (Dole, Canada)	46	250 g	34	15
Plum, raw, NS (Canada)	24	120 g	14	3
Plum, raw, NS (Italy)	53	120 g	11	6
Average of two studies	39	120 g	12	5

* Average

FOOD	GI	NOMINAL SERVE SIZE	AVAILABLE CARB PER SERVE	GL PER SERVE
Prunes, pitted (Sunsweet, USA)	29	60 g	33	10
Raisins (Canada)	64	60 g	44	28
Rockmelon/Cantaloupe, raw (Australia)	65	120 g	6	4
Strawberries, fresh, raw (Australia)	40	120 g	3	1
Strawberry jam	51	30 g	20	10
Strawberry Real Fruit Bars (Uncle Toby's, Australia)	90	30 g	26	23
Sultanas	56	60 g	45	25
Tomato juice, no added sugar (Berri, Australia)	38	250 g	9	4
Tropical Fruity Bitz™, (Blackmores, Australia)	41	15 g	11	5
Vitari, wild berry, non-dairy, frozen dessert (Nestlé, Australia)	59	100 g	21	12
Watermelon, raw (Australia)	72	120 g	6	4
Wild Berry Fruity Bitz™ (Blackmores, Australia)	35	15 g	12	4

INFANT FORMULA AND WEANING FOODS

Formula

FOOD	GI	NOMINAL SERVE SIZE	AVAILABLE CARB PER SERVE	GL PER SERVE
Infasoy™, soy-based, milk-free (Wyeth, Australia)	55	100 ml	7	4
Karicare™ formula with omega oils (Nutricia, New Zealand)	35	100 ml	7	2
Nan-1™ infant formula with iron (Nestlé, Australia)	30	100 ml	8	2
S-26™ infant formula (Wyeth, Australia)	36	100 ml	7	3

* Average

FOOD	GI	NOMINAL SERVE SIZE	AVAILABLE CARB PER SERVE	GL PER SERVE
Weaning Foods				
Farex™ baby rice (Heinz, Australia)	95	87 g	6	6
Robinsons First Tastes from 4 months (Nutricia, UK)				
Apple, apricot and banana cereal	56	75 g	13	7
Creamed porridge	59	75 g	9	5
Rice pudding	59	75 g	11	6
Heinz for Baby from 4 months (Heinz, Australia)				
Chicken and noodles with vegetables, strained	67	120 g	7	5
Sweetcorn and rice	65	120 g	15	10

LEGUMES AND NUTS

FOOD	GI	NOMINAL SERVE SIZE	AVAILABLE CARB PER SERVE	GL PER SERVE
Baked Beans				
Baked Beans, canned (Canada)	40			
Baked Beans, canned beans in tomato sauce (Libby, Canada)	56			
Average of two studies	48	150 g	17	8
Beans, dried, boiled				
Beans, dried, type NS (Italy)	36	150 g	30	11
Beans, dried, type NS (Italy)	20	150 g	30	6
Average of two studies	29	150 g	30	9
Blackeyed beans/peas (Cowpeas), boiled				
Blackeyed beans (Canada)	50	150 g	21	11
Blackeyed beans (Canada)	33	150 g	21	7
Average of two studies	42	150 g	21	9
Butter Beans				
Butter beans (South Africa)	28	150 g	20	5

* Average

FOOD	GI	NOMINAL SERVE SIZE	AVAILABLE CARB PER SERVE	GL PER SERVE
Butter beans, dried, cooked (South Africa)	29	150 g	20	6
Butter beans (Canada)	36	150 g	20	7
Average of three studies	31	150 g	20	6
Butter beans, dried, boiled + 5g sucrose (South Africa)	30	150 g	20	6
Butter beans, dried, boiled + 10g sucrose (South Africa)	31	150 g	20	6
Butter beans, dried, boiled + 15g sucrose (South Africa)	54	150 g	20	11
Chickpeas (Garbanzo beans, Bengal gram), boiled				
Chickpeas (Cicer arietinum Linn), boiled (Philippines)	10	150 g	24	2
Chickpeas, dried, boiled (Canada)	31	150 g	24	7
Chickpeas (Canada)	35*	150 g	24	8
Average of three studies	25	150 g	24	6
Chickpeas, canned in brine (Lancia-Bravo, Canada)	42	150 g	22	9
Chickpeas, curry, canned (Canasia, Canada)	41	150 g	16	7
Haricot/navy beans				
Haricot/navy beans, pressure cooked (King Grains, Canada)	29	150 g	33	9
Haricot/navy beans, dried, boiled (Canada)	30	150 g	30	9
Haricot/navy beans, boiled (Canada)	31	150 g	30	9
Haricot/navy beans (King Grains, Canada)	39	150 g	30	12
Haricot/navy beans, pressure cooked (King Grains, Canada)	59	150 g	33	19
Average of five studies	38	150 g	31	12

* Average

FOOD	GI	NOMINAL SERVE SIZE	AVAILABLE CARB PER SERVE	GL PER SERVE
Kidney Beans				
Kidney/white bean (Phaseolus vulgaris Linn), boiled (Philippines)	13	150 g	25	3
Kidney beans (Phaseolus vulgaris) (India)	19	150 g	25	5
Kidney beans (USA)	23	150 g	25	6
Kidney beans, dried, boiled (France)	23	150 g	25	6
Kidney beans (Phaseolus vulgaris L.), red, boiled (Sweden)	25	150 g	25	6
Kidney beans (Canada)	29	150 g	25	7
Kidney beans, dried, boiled (Canada)	42	150 g	25	10
Kidney beans (Canada)	46	150 g	25	11
mean of eight studies	28	150 g	25	7
Kidney beans (Phaseolus vulgaris L.) – autoclaved	34	150 g	25	8
Kidney beans, canned (Lancia-Bravo, Canada)	52	150 g	17	9
Kidney beans, soaked 12 h, stored moist 24 h, steamed 1 h (India)	70	150 g	25	17
Lentils, type NS				
Lentils, type NS (USA)	28			
Lentils, type NS (Canada)	29			
Average of two studies	29	150 g	18	5
Lentils, green				
Lentils, green, dried, boiled (Canada)	22	150 g	18	4
Lentils, green, dried, boiled (France)	30	150 g	18	6
Lentils, green, dried, boiled (Australia)	37	150 g	14	5
Average of three studies	30	150 g	17	5
Lentils, green, canned in brine (Lancia-Bravo Foods Ltd., Canada)	52	150 g	17	9

* Average

FOOD	GI	NOMINAL SERVE SIZE	AVAILABLE CARB PER SERVE	GL PER SERVE
Lentils, red				
Lentils, red, dried, boiled (Canada)	18	150 g	18	3
Lentils, red, dried, boiled (Canada)	21	150 g	18	4
Lentils, red, dried, boiled (Canada)	31	150 g	18	6
Lentils, red, dried, boiled (Canada)	32	150 g	18	6
Average of four studies	26	150 g	18	5
Lima beans				
Lima beans, baby, frozen (York, Canada)	32	150 g	30	10
Marrowfat peas				
Marrowfat peas, dried, boiled (USA)	31			
Marrowfat peas, dried, boiled (Canada)	47			
Average of two studies	39	150 g	19	7
Mung beans				
Mung bean (Phaseolus areus Roxb), boiled (Philippines)	31	150 g	17	5
Mung bean, fried (Australia)	53			
Mung bean, germinated (Australia)	25	150 g	17	4
Mung bean, pressure cooked (Australia)	42	150 g	17	7
Pinto beans				
Pinto beans, boiled (Canada)	39	150 g	26	10
Pinto beans, canned in brine (Lancia-Bravo, Canada)	45	150 g	22	10
Romano beans (Canada)	46	150 g	18	8
Soy beans				
Soy beans, boiled (Canada)	15	150 g	6	1
Soy beans, boiled (Australia)	20	150 g	6	1
Average of two studies	18	150 g	6	1
Soy beans, canned (Canada)	14	150 g	6	1

* Average

FOOD	GI	NOMINAL SERVE SIZE	AVAILABLE CARB PER SERVE	GL PER SERVE
MEAL REPLACEMENT PRODUCTS				
Hazelnut and Apricot bar (Dietworks, Australia)	42	50 g	22	9
L.E.A.N™ products (Usana, USA)				
L.E.A.N Fibergy™ bar, Harvest Oat	45	50 g	29	13
Nutrimeal™, drink powder, Dutch Chocolate	26	250 g	13	3
L.E.A.N (Life long) Nutribar™, Peanut Crunch	30	40 g	19	6
L.E.A.N (Life long) Nutribar™, Chocolate Crunch	32	40 g	19	6
Average of two Nutribars	31	40 g	19	6
Worldwide Sport Nutrition low-carbohydrate products (USA)				
Designer chocolate, sugar-free	14	35 g	22	3
Burn-it™ bars				
Chocolate deluxe	29	50 g	8	2
Peanut butter	23	50 g	6	1
Pure-protein™ bars				
Chewy choc-chip	30	80 g	14	4
Chocolate deluxe	38	80 g	13	5
Peanut butter	22	80 g	9	2
Strawberry shortcake	43	80 g	13	6
White chocolate mousse	40	80 g	15	6
Pure-protein™ cookies				
Choc-chip cookie dough	25	55 g	11	3
Coconut	42	55 g	9	4
Peanut butter	37	55 g	9	3

* Average

FOOD	GI	NOMINAL SERVE SIZE	AVAILABLE CARB PER SERVE	GL PER SERVE
MIXED MEALS AND CONVENIENCE FOODS				
Chicken nuggets, frozen, reheated (Australia)	46	100 g	16	7
Fish Fingers (Canada)	38	100 g	19	7
Fish fillet, reduced fat, crumbed (Maggi)	43	85 g	16	7
Greek lentil stew with a bread roll, home made (Australia)	40	360 g	37	15
Kugel (Polish dish containing egg noodles, sugar, cheese and raisins) (Israel)	65	150 g	48	31
Lean Cuisine™, chicken with rice (Nestlé, Australia)	36	400 g	68	24
Pies, beef, party size (Farmland, Australia)	45	100 g	27	12
Pizza, cheese (Pillsbury, Canada)	60	100 g	27	16
Pizza, plain (Italy)	80	100 g	27	22
Pizza, Super Supreme, pan (Pizza Hut, Australia)	36	100 g	24	9
Pizza, Super Supreme, thin and crispy (Pizza Hut, Australia)	30	100 g	22	7
Pizza, Vegetarian Supreme, thin and crispy (Pizza Hut, Australia)	49	100 g	25	12
Sausages NS (Canada)	28	100 g	3	1
Sirloin chop with mixed vegetables and mashed potato (Australia)	66	360 g	53	35
Spaghetti bolognaise, home made (Australia)	52	360 g	48	25
Stirfried vegetables with chicken and rice, home made (Australia)	73	360 g	75	55

* Average

FOOD	GI	NOMINAL SERVE SIZE	AVAILABLE CARB PER SERVE	GL PER SERVE
Sushi, salmon (Australia)	48	100 g	36	17
Sushi, roasted sea algae, vinegar and rice (Japan)	55	100 g	37	20
Average of two studies	52	100 g	37	19
Tuna pattie, reduced fat (Maggi)	45	84 g	17	8
White boiled rice, grilled beefburger, cheese, and butter (France)	27	440 g	50	14
White boiled rice, grilled beefburger, cheese and butter (France)	22	440 g	50	11
Average in two groups of subjects	25	440 g	50	13
White bread with toppings				
White bread, butter, regular cow's milk cheese and fresh cucumber (Sweden)	55	200 g	68	38
White bread, butter, yoghurt and pickled cucumber (Sweden)	39	200 g	28	11
White bread with butter (Canada)	59	100 g	48	29
White bread with skim milk cheese (Canada)	55	100 g	47	26
White bread with butter and skim milk cheese (Canada)	62	100 g	38	23
White/wholemeal bread with peanut butter (Canada)	51	100 g	44	23
White/wholemeal bread with peanut butter (Canada)	67	100 g	44	30
Average of two studies	59	100 g	44	26

NUTS

Cashew nuts, salted (Coles Supermarkets, Australia)	22	50 g	13	3
Pecans, raw	10	50 g	3	0
Peanuts, crushed (South Africa)	7	50 g	4	0

* Average

FOOD	GI	NOMINAL SERVE SIZE	AVAILABLE CARB PER SERVE	GL PER SERVE
Peanuts (Canada)	13	50 g	7	1
Peanuts (Mexico)	23	50 g	7	2
Average of three studies	14	50 g	6	1

NUTRITIONAL SUPPORT PRODUCTS

FOOD	GI	NOMINAL SERVE SIZE	AVAILABLE CARB PER SERVE	GL PER SERVE
Choice dm™, vanilla (Mead Johnson, USA)	23	237 ml	24	6
Enercal Plus™ (Wyeth-Ayerst, USA)	61	237 ml	40	24
Enrich Plus™ shake, vanilla	58	200 ml	40	23
Ensure™ (Abbott, Australia)	50	237 ml	40	19
Ensure™, vanilla (Abbott, Australia)	48	250 ml	34	16
Ensure™ bar, chocolate fudge brownie (Abbott, Australia) *	43	38 g	20	8
Ensure Plus™, vanilla (Abbott, Australia)	40	237 ml	47	19
Ensure Pudding™, vanilla (Abbott, USA)	36	113 g	26	9
Glucerna™ bar, lemon crunch	27	38 g	20	5
Glucerna™ SR shake, vanilla	19	230 ml	24	5
Glucerna™, vanilla (Abbott, USA)	31	237 ml	23	7
Jevity™ (Abbott, Australia)	48	237 ml	36	17
Resource Diabetic™, vanilla (Novartis, USA)	34	237 ml	23	8
Resource Diabetic™, chocolate (Novartis, New Zealand)	16	237 ml	41	7
Resource™ thickened orange juice (Novartis, New Zealand)	47	237 ml	39	18
Resource™ thickened orange juice (Novartis, New Zealand)	54	237 ml	36	19
Resource™ fruit beverage, peach flavour (Novartis, New Zealand)	40	237 ml	41	16

* Average

FOOD	GI	NOMINAL SERVE SIZE	AVAILABLE CARB PER SERVE	GL PER SERVE
Resource Plus, chocolate	43	237 ml	52	22
Sustagen™, Dutch Chocolate (Mead Johnson, Australia)	31	250 ml	41	13
Sustagen™ Hospital with extra fibre (Mead Johnson, Australia)	33	250 ml	44	15
Sustagen™ Instant Pudding, vanilla (Mead Johnson, Australia)	27	250 g	47	13
Ultracal™ with fiber (Mead Johnson, USA)	40	237 ml	29	12

PASTA and NOODLES

FOOD	GI	NOMINAL SERVE SIZE	AVAILABLE CARB PER SERVE	GL PER SERVE
Capellini (Primo, Canada)	45	180 g	45	20
Corn pasta, gluten-free (Orgran, Australia)	78	180 g	42	32
Fettucine, egg				
Fettucine, egg	32	180 g	46	15
Fettucine, egg (Mother Earth, Australia)	47	180 g	46	22
Average of two studies	40	180 g	46	18
Gnocchi				
Gnocchi, NS (Latina, Australia)	68	180 g	48	33
Instant noodles				
Instant 'two-minute' noodles, Maggi® (Australia)	46			
Instant 'two-minute' noodles, Maggi® (New Zealand)	48			
Instant noodles (Mr Noodle, Canada)	47			
Average of three studies	47	180 g	40	19

* Average

FOOD	GI	NOMINAL SERVE SIZE	AVAILABLE CARB PER SERVE	GL PER SERVE
Linguine				
Thick, durum wheat, white, fresh (Sweden)	43	180 g	48	21
Thick, fresh, durum wheat flour (Sweden)	48	180 g	48	23
Average of two studies	46	180 g	48	22
Thin, durum wheat (Sweden)	49	180 g	48	23
Thin, fresh, durum wheat flour (Sweden)	61	180 g	48	29
Average of four studies	52	180 g	45	23
Mung bean noodles				
Lungkow beanthread noodles (National Cereals, China)	26	180 g	45	12
Mung bean noodles (Longkou beanthread) (Yantai, China)	39	180 g	45	18
Average of two studies	33			
Macaroni				
Macaroni, plain, boiled 5 min (Lancia-Bravo, Canada)	45	180 g	49	22
Macaroni, plain, boiled (Turkey)	48	180 g	49	23
Average of two studies	47	180 g	48	23
Macaroni and Cheese, boxed (Kraft, Canada)	64	180 g	51	32
Ravioli				
Ravioli (Australia)	39	180 g	38	15
Rice noodles/pasta				
Rice noodles, dried, boiled (Thai World, Thailand)	61	180 g	39	23
Rice noodles, freshly made, boiled (Sydney, Australia)	40	180 g	39	15

* Average

FOOD	GI	NOMINAL SERVE SIZE	AVAILABLE CARB PER SERVE	GL PER SERVE
Rice pasta, brown, boiled 16 min (Rice Growers, Australia)	92	180 g	38	35
Rice and maize pasta, gluten-free, Ris'O'Mais (Orgran, Australia)	76	180 g	49	37
Rice vermicelli, Kongmoon (China)	58	180 g	39	22
Spaghetti				
Spaghetti, gluten-free, canned in tomato sauce (Orgran, Australia)	68	220 g	27	19
Spaghetti, protein enriched, boiled 7 min (Catelli, Canada)	27	180 g	52	14
Spaghetti, white, boiled 5 min				
Boiled 5 min (Lancia-Bravo, Canada)	32	180 g	48	15
Boiled 5 min (Canada)	37*	180 g	48	18
Boiled 5 min (Middle East)	44	180 g	48	21
Average of three studies	38	180 g	48	18
Spaghetti, white or type NS, boiled 10-15 min				
White, durum wheat, boiled 10 min (Barilla, Italy)	58	180 g	48	28
White, durum wheat flour, boiled 12 min (Starhushålls, Sweden)	47	180 g	48	23
White, durum wheat flour, boiled 12 min (Sweden)	53	180 g	48	25
Boiled 15 min (Lancia-Bravo, Canada)	32	180 g	48	15
Boiled 15 min (Lancia-Bravo, Canada)				
Boiled 15 min (Canada)	41	180 g	48	20
White, boiled 15 min in salted water (Unico, Canada)	44	180 g	48	21
Average of seven studies	44	180 g	48	21

---

* Average

FOOD	GI	NOMINAL SERVE SIZE	AVAILABLE CARB PER SERVE	GL PER SERVE
Spaghetti, white or type NS, boiled 20 min				
White, durum wheat, boiled 20 min (Australia)	58	180 g	44	26
Durum wheat, boiled 20 min (USA)	64	180 g	43	27
Average of two studies	61	180 g	44	27
Spaghetti, white, boiled				
White (Denmark)	33	180 g	48	16
White, durum wheat (Catelli, Canada)	34	180 g	48	16
White (Australia)	38	180 g	44	17
White (Canada)	47*	180 g	48	23
White (Vetta, Australia)	49	180 g	44	22
Average of five studies	42	180 g	47	20
Spaghetti, white, durum wheat semolina (Panzani, France)				
Boiled for 11 min	59	180 g	48	28
Boiled for 16.5 min	65	180 g	48	31
Boiled for 22 min	46	180 g	48	22
Average of three cooking times	57	180 g	48	27
Spaghetti, wholemeal, boiled				
Wholemeal (USA)	32	180 g	44	14
Wholemeal (Canada)	42	180 g	40	17
Average of two studies	37	180 g	42	16
Spirali				
Spirali, durum wheat, white, boiled (Vetta, Australia)	43	180 g	44	19
Tortellini				
Tortellini, cheese (Stouffer, Canada)	50	180 g	21	10
Udon noodles				

* Average

FOOD	GI	NOMINAL SERVE SIZE	AVAILABLE CARB PER SERVE	GL PER SERVE
Udon noodles, plain, reheated 5 min (Australia)	62	180 g	48	30
Vermicelli				
Vermicelli, white, boiled (Australia)	35	180 g	44	16

PROTEIN FOODS

FOOD	GI	NOMINAL SERVE SIZE	AVAILABLE CARB PER SERVE	GL PER SERVE
Beef	[0]	120 g	0	0
Cheese	[0]	120 g	0	0
Eggs	[0]	120 g	0	0
Fish	[0]	120 g	0	0
Lamb	[0]	120 g	0	0
Pork	[0]	120 g	0	0
Salami	[0]	120 g	0	0
Shellfish (prawns, crab, lobster etc)	[0]	120 g	0	0
Tuna	[0]	120 g	0	0
Veal	[0]	120 g	0	0

SNACK FOODS AND CONFECTIONERY

FOOD	GI	NOMINAL SERVE SIZE	AVAILABLE CARB PER SERVE	GL PER SERVE
Burger Rings™ (Smith's, Australia)	90	50 g	31	28
Chocolate, milk, plain with sucrose (Belgium)	34	50 g	22	7
Chocolate, milk (Cadbury's, Australia)	49	50 g	30	14
Chocolate, milk, Dove® (Mars, Australia)	45	50 g	30	13
Chocolate, milk (Nestlé, Australia)	42	50 g	31	13
Average of four studies	43	50 g	28	12
Chocolate, milk, plain, low-sugar with maltitol (Belgium)	35	50 g	22	8
Chocolate, white, Milky Bar® (Nestlé, Australia)	44	50 g	29	13

* Average

FOOD	GI	NOMINAL SERVE SIZE	AVAILABLE CARB PER SERVE	GL PER SERVE
Corn chips, plain, salted (Doritos™, Australia)	42	50 g	25	11
Corn chips, Nachips™ (Old El Paso, Canada)	74	50 g	29	21
Average of three studies	63	50 g	26	17
Fruit bar apricot filled (Mother Earth, New Zealand)	50	50 g	34	17
Fruit Fingers Heinz Kidz™, banana (Heinz, Australia)	61	30 g	20	12
Fruity Bitz™, apricot (Blackmores, Australia)	42	15 g	12	5
Fruity Bitz™, berry (Blackmores, Australia)	35	15 g	12	4
Fruity Bitz™, tropical (Blackmores, Australia)	41	15 g	11	5
Average of three flavours	39	15 g	12	4
Jelly beans, assorted colors (Australia)	78*	30 g	28	22
Kudos Whole Grain Bars, chocolate chip (USA)	62	50 g	32	20
Life Savers®, peppermint candy (Nestlé, Australia)	70	30 g	30	21
M & M's®, peanut (Australia)	33	30 g	17	6
Mars Bar® (Australia)	62	60 g	40	25
Mars Bar® (USA)	68	60 g	40	27
Average of two studies	65	60 g	40	26
Muesli bar containing dried fruit (Uncle Toby's, Australia)	61	30 g	21	13
Nougat, Jijona (La Fama, Spain)	32	30 g	12	4
Nutella®, chocolate hazelnut spread (Australia)	33	20 g	12	4

* Average

FOOD	GI	NOMINAL SERVE SIZE	AVAILABLE CARB PER SERVE	GL PER SERVE
Nuts, cashew salted (Coles Supermarkets, Australia)	22	50 g	13	3
Peanuts, crushed (South Africa)	7	50 g	4	0
Peanuts (Canada)	13	50 g	7	1
Peanuts (Mexico)	23	50 g	7	2
Average of three studies	14	50 g	6	1
Pecan				
Popcorn, plain, cooked in microwave oven (Green's, Australia)	55	20 g	11	6
Popcorn, plain, cooked in microwave oven (Uncle Toby's, Australia)	89	20 g	11	10
Average of two studies	72	20 g	11	8
Pop Tarts™, double choc (Kellogg's, Australia)	70	50 g	35	24
Potato crisps, plain, salted (Arnott's, Australia)	57	50 g	18	10
Potato crisps, plain, salted (Canada)	51	50 g	24	12
Average of two studies	54	50 g	21	11
Pretzels, (Parker's, Australia)	83	30 g	20	16
Real Fruit Bars, strawberry (Uncle Toby's, Australia)	90	30 g	26	23
Roll-Ups® (Uncle Toby's, Australia)	99	30 g	25	24
Skittles® (Australia)	70	50 g	45	32
Snack bar, Apple Cinnamon (Con Agra, USA)	40	50 g	29	12
Snack bar, Peanut Butter & Choc-Chip (USA)	37	50 g	27	10
Snickers Bar® (Australia)	41	60 g	36	15
Snickers Bar® (USA)	68	60 g	34	23
Average of two studies	55	60 g	35	19
Sunripe school straps	40	15 g	11	4
Twisties™ cheese (Smith's, Australia)	74	50 g	29	22

* Average

FOOD	GI	NOMINAL SERVE SIZE	AVAILABLE CARB PER SERVE	GL PER SERVE
Twix® Cookie Bar, caramel (USA)	44	60 g	39	17

SPORTS BARS

FOOD	GI	NOMINAL SERVE SIZE	AVAILABLE CARB PER SERVE	GL PER SERVE
Power Bar®, chocolate (USA)	56*	65 g	42	24
Ironman PR bar®, chocolate (USA)	39	65 g	26	10

SOUPS

FOOD	GI	NOMINAL SERVE SIZE	AVAILABLE CARB PER SERVE	GL PER SERVE
Black Bean (Wil-Pack, USA)	64	250 ml	27	17
Green Pea, canned (Campbell's, Canada)	66	250 ml	41	27
Lentil, canned (Unico, Canada)	44	250 ml	21	9
Minestrone, Country Ladle™ (Campbell's, Australia)	39	250 ml	18	7
Noodle soup (Turkish soup with stock and noodles)	1	250 ml	9	0
Split Pea (Wil-Pak, USA)	60	250 ml	27	16
Tarhana soup (Turkish soup)	20			
Tomato soup (Canada)	38	250 ml	17	6

SUGARS

Blue Agave cactus nectar, high-fructose

FOOD	GI	NOMINAL SERVE SIZE	AVAILABLE CARB PER SERVE	GL PER SERVE
Organic Agave Cactus Nectar, light, 90% fructose (Western Commerce, USA)	11	10 g	8	1
Organic Agave Cactus Nectar, light, 97% fructose (Western Commerce, USA)	10	10 g	8	1

Fructose

FOOD	GI	NOMINAL SERVE SIZE	AVAILABLE CARB PER SERVE	GL PER SERVE
25g portion (Canada)	11			
50g portion (Canada)	12			
50g portion	20			

* Average

FOOD	GI	NOMINAL SERVE SIZE	AVAILABLE CARB PER SERVE	GL PER SERVE
50g portion	21			
50g portion (USA)	24			
25g portion, fed with oats	25			
Average of six studies	19	10 g	10	2
Glucose				
Dextrose	100	10 g	10	10
Glucose consumed with 3 g American ginseng	78	10 g	10	8
Glucose consumed with gum/fibre				
15 g apple and orange fibre (FITA, Australia)	79	10 g	8	6
14.5 g guar gum	62	10 g	10	6
14.5 g oat gum (78% oat ß-glucan)	57	10 g	10	6
20 g acacia gum	85	10 g	10	9
Honey				
Locust honey (Romania)	32	25 g	21	7
Yellow box (Australia)	35	25 g	18	6
Stringy Bark (Australia)	44	25 g	21	9
Red Gum (Australia)	46	25 g	18	8
Iron Bark (Australia)	48	25 g	15	7
Yapunya (Australia)	52	25 g	17	9
Pure (Capilano, Australia)	58	25 g	21	12
Commercial Blend (Australia)	62	25 g	18	11
Salvation Jane (Australia)	64	25 g	15	10
Commercial Blend (Australia)	72	25 g	13	9
Honey NS (Canada)	87	25 g	21	18
Average of 11 types of honey	55	25 g	18	10
Lactose				
Lactose	46	10 g	10	5
Maltose				
Maltose	105	10 g	10	11

* Average

FOOD	GI	NOMINAL SERVE SIZE	AVAILABLE CARB PER SERVE	GL PER SERVE
Sucrose				
Sucrose	61	10 g	10	6

VEGETABLES

FOOD	GI	NOMINAL SERVE SIZE	AVAILABLE CARB PER SERVE	GL PER SERVE
Artichokes	[0]	80 g	0	0
Avocado	[0]	80 g	0	0
Beetroot	64	80 g	7	5
Bokchoy	[0]	80 g	0	0
Broad beans	79	80 g	11	9
Broccoli	[0]	80 g	0	0
Cabbage	[0]	80 g	0	0
Carrots, peeled, boiled (Australia)	49	80 g	5	2
Cassava, boiled, with salt (Kenya, Africa)	46	100 g	27	12
Capsicum	[0]	80 g	0	0
Cauliflower	[0]	80 g	0	0
Celery	[0]	80 g	0	0
Corn, sweet, 'Honey & Pearl' variety (New Zealand)	37	80 g	16	6
Corn, sweet, on the cob, boiled (Australia)	48	80 g	16	8
Corn, sweet, (Canada)	59	80 g	18	11
Corn, sweet, boiled (USA)	60	80 g	18	11
Corn, sweet, (South Africa)	62	80 g	18	11
Average of five studies	54	80 g	17	9
Corn, sweet, diet-pack, (USA)	46	80 g	14	7
Corn, sweet, frozen (Canada)	47	80 g	15	7
Cucumber	[0]	80 g	0	0
French beans (runner beans)	[0]	80 g	0	0
Leafy vegetables (spinach, rocket etc)	[0]	80 g	0	0
Lettuce	[0]	80 g	0	0

* Average

FOOD	GI	NOMINAL SERVE SIZE	AVAILABLE CARB PER SERVE	GL PER SERVE
Parsnips	97	80 g	12	12
Peas, frozen, boiled (Canada)	39	80 g	7	3
Peas, frozen, boiled (Canada)	51	80 g	7	4
Peas, green (*Pisum sativum*) (India)	54	80 g	7	4
Average of three studies	48	80 g	7	3
Potato baked				
Ontario, white, baked in skin (Canada)	60	150 g	30	18
Potato, baked, Russet Burbank				
Russet, baked without fat (Canada)	56			
Russet, baked without fat, 45–60 min (USA)	78			
Russet, baked without fat (USA)	94			
Russet, baked without fat (USA)	111			
Average of four studies	85	150 g	30	26
Potato boiled				
Desiree (Australia)	101	150 g	17	17
Nardine (New Zealand)	70	150 g	25	18
Ontario (Canada)	58	150 g	27	16
Pontiac (Australia)	88	150 g	18	16
Prince Edward Island (Canada)	63	150 g	18	11
Sebago (Australia)	87	150 g	17	14
White (Romania)	41	150 g	30	12
White (Canada)	54	150 g	27	15
Type NS (India)	76	150 g	34	26
Type NS refrigerated, reheated (India)	23	150 g	34	8
Potato canned				
Prince Edward Island (Cobi Foods, Canada)	61	150 g	18	11

* Average

FOOD	GI	NOMINAL SERVE SIZE	AVAILABLE CARB PER SERVE	GL PER SERVE
New (Mint Tiny Taters Edgell's, Australia)	65	150 g	18	12
Average of two studies	63	150 g	18	11
Potato, French fries				
French fries, frozen and reheated (Cavendish Farms, Canada)	75	150 g	29	22
Potato instant mashed				
Instant (France)	74			
Instant (Canada)	84*			
Instant (Edgell's, Australia)	86			
Instant (Carnation, Canada)	86			
Instant (USA)	97			
Average of six studies	85	150 g	20	17
Potato, mashed				
Type NS (Canada)	67			
Type NS (South Africa)	71			
Type NS (France)	83			
Prince Edward Island, (Canada)	73	150 g	18	13
Pontiac (Australia)	91	150 g	20	18
Average of five studies	92	150 g	20	18
Potato microwaved				
Pontiac, peeled and microwaved on high for 6–7.5 min (Australia)	79	150 g	18	14
Type NS, microwaved (USA)	82	150 g	33	27
Potato new				
New (Canada)	47			
New (Canada)	54			
New (Canada)	70			
New (Australia)	78			
Average of four studies	62	150 g	21	13

* Average

FOOD	GI	NOMINAL SERVE SIZE	AVAILABLE CARB PER SERVE	GL PER SERVE
Potato steamed				
Potato, peeled, steamed (India)	65	150 g	27	18
Potato dumplings (Italy)	52	150 g	45	24
Potato sweet				
Sweet potato, *Ipomoea batatas* (Australia)	44	150 g	25	11
Sweet potato, (Canada)	48	150 g	34	16
Sweet potato (Canada)	59	150 g	30	18
Sweet potato, kumara (New Zealand)	78	150 g	25	20
Average of five studies	61	150 g	28	17
Pumpkin				
Pumpkin (South Africa)	75	80 g	4	3
Squash				
Squash	[0]	80 g	0	0
Swede				
Swede (rutabaga) (Canada)	72	150 g	10	7
Tapioca				
Tapioca boiled with milk (General Mills, Canada)	81	250 g	18	14
Tapioca (*Manihot utilissima*), steamed one hour (India)	70	250 g	18	12
Taro				
Taro (*Colocasia esculenta*), boiled (Australia)	54			
Taro, boiled (New Zealand)	56			
Average of two studies	55	150 g	8	4
Yam				
Yam, peeled, boiled (New Zealand)	25			
Yam, peeled, boiled (New Zealand)	35			
Yam (Canada)	51			
Average of three studies	37	150 g	36	13

* Average

LOW TO HIGH
GI VALUES

For those people who wish to choose the lowest GI diet possible we've created the following listing in order of GI, ie from lowest to highest. It is also divided into food categories, so that when you want to find a low GI vegetable or a low GI fruit, for example, the information is at your fingertips. This listing may also provide you with new food ideas to try, rather than just checking the GI value of the food you eat.

We have still included some medium and high GI foods as well. As we discuss in *The New Glucose Revolution* you don't need to eat all your carbohydrate from low GI sources. If half of your carbohydrate is from low GI sources you are doing well. If you eat a low GI food at each meal, then your overall GI will be reduced.

Don't forget either that the glycaemic load is also included in these lists. In this way you can choose foods with either a low GI and/or a low GL. But don't make the mistake of using GL alone. If you do, you might find yourself eating a diet with very little carbohydrate but a lot of fat, especially saturated fat, and excessive amounts of protein.

FOOD	GI	NOMINAL SERVE SIZE	AVAILABLE CARB PER SERVE	GL PER SERVE
Biscuits				
Snack Right™ Fruit Slice	48	25 g	19	9
Highland Oatmeal™	55	25 g	18	10
Digestives	59*	25 g	16	10
Shredded Wheatmeal™	62	25 g	18	11
Shortbread	64	25 g	16	10
Milk Arrowroot™	69	25 g	18	12
Morning Coffee™	79	25 g	19	15
Bread				
Bürgen® Soy-Lin	36	30 g	9	3
Performax™ (Country Life)	38	30 g	13	5
9-Grain Multi-Grain (Tip Top)	43	30 g	14	11
Bürgen™ Fruit loaf	44	30 g	13	6
Continental fruit loaf	47	30 g	15	7
Ploughman's™ Wholegrain	47	30 g	14	7
Bürgen® Oat Bran & Honey bread	49	40 g	13	7
Bürgen™ Dark/Swiss rye	65	30 g	10	9
Sourdough rye	53	30 g	12	6
Fruit and Spice Loaf (Buttercup)	54	30 g	15	8
Multigrain Spelt wheat Loaf	54	30 g	15	8
Sourdough wheat	54	30 g	14	8
Spelt multigrain bread	54	30 g	12	7
Vogel's Honey & Oats	55	30 g	14	7
Pita bread	57	30 g	17	10
Sunflower and barley bread (Riga)	57	30 g	11	6
Wholemeal rye bread	58*	30 g	14	8
Roggenbrot, (Vogel's)	59	30 g	14	8
Hamburger bun, white	61	30 g	15	9

* Average

FOOD	GI	NOMINAL SERVE SIZE	AVAILABLE CARB PER SERVE	GL PER SERVE
Rice bread, high-amylose Doongara rice	61	30 g	12	7
Pain au lait	63	60 g	32	20
Ploughman's™ wholemeal	64	30 g	13	9
Barley flour bread	67	30 g	13	9
Helga's™ Classic Seed Loaf	68	30 g	14	9
Helga's™ traditional wholemeal bread	70	30 g	13	9
Melba toast	70	30 g	23	16
White bread	70	30 g	14	10
Bagel, white	72	70 g	35	25
Rice bread, low-amylose Calrose rice	72	30 g	12	8
Kaiser rolls	73	30 g	16	12
Lebanese bread, white	75	30 g	16	12
Blackbread (Riga)	76	30 g	13	10
Wholemeal bread	77	30 g	12	9
Gluten-free multigrain bread	79	30 g	13	10
Wonderwhite™ (Buttercup)	80	30 g	14	11
Schinkenbrot (Riga)	86	30 g	14	12
Baguette, white	95	30 g	15	14
Breakfast bars				
Fruity-Bix™ bar, wild berry	51	30 g	19	9
Fruity-Bix™ bar, fruit and nut	56	30 g	19	10
Sustain™ bar	57	30 g	25	14
Rice Bubble Treat™ bar	63	30 g	24	15
Crunchy Nut Cornflakes™ bar	72	30 g	26	19
K-Time Just Right™ bar	72	30 g	24	17
K-Time Strawberry Crunch™ bar	77	30 g	25	19
Fibre Plus™ bar	78	30 g	23	18

* Average

FOOD	GI	NOMINAL SERVE SIZE	AVAILABLE CARB PER SERVE	GL PER SERVE
Breakfast cereal				
Rice Bran, extruded	19	30 g	14	3
All-Bran™	30	30 g	15	5
All-Bran Soy 'n' Fibre™	33	30 g	14	4
Guardian™	37	30 g	12	5
All-Bran Fruit 'n' Oats™	39	30 g	17	7
Muesli, gluten-free	39	30 g	19	7
Ultra-bran™, soy and linseed	41	30 g	13	5
Muesli, toasted (Purina)	43	30 g	17	7
Healthwise™ for heart health	48	30 g	19	9
Komplete™	48	30 g	21	10
Muesli, Natural	48*	30 g	18	8
Soytana™ (Vogel's)	49	45 g	25	12
Traditional porridge oats	51	250 g	21	11
Special K™	54	30 g	21	11
Frosties™	55	30 g	26	15
Porridge, made from whole rolled oats	55*	250 g	21	11
Hi-Bran Weet-Bix™ with soy and linseed	57	30 g	16	9
Oat bran Weet-Bix™	57	30 g	20	11
Mini Wheats™, whole wheat	58	30 g	21	12
Just Right™	60	30 g	22	13
Soy Tasty™	60	30 g	20	12
Hi-Bran Weet-Bix™	61	30 g	17	10
Just Right Just Grains™	62	30 g	23	14
Sultana Goldies™	65	30 g	21	13
Healthwise™ for bowel health	66	30 g	18	12
Instant porridge	66	250 g	26	17
Nutrigrain™	66*	30 g	15	10

* Average

FOOD	GI	NOMINAL SERVE SIZE	AVAILABLE CARB PER SERVE	GL PER SERVE
Good Start™, muesli wheat biscuits	68	30 g	20	14
Vita-Brits™	68	30 g	20	13
Sustain™	68	30 g	22	15
Froot Loops™	69	30 g	26	18
Weet-Bix™	69	30 g	17	12
Lite-Bix™, no added sugar	70	30 g	20	14
Pop Tarts™, chocolate	70	50 g	36	25
Whole wheat Goldies™	70	30 g	20	14
Golden Wheats™	71	30 g	23	16
Honey Smacks™	71	30 g	23	16
Cornflakes, Crunchy Nut™	72	30 g	24	17
Honey Goldies™	72	30 g	21	15
Mini Wheats™, blackcurrant	72	30 g	21	15
Wheat-bites™	72	30 g	25	18
Sultana Bran™	73	30 g	19	14
Bran Flakes™	74	30 g	18	13
Shredded Wheat	75	30 g	20	15
Coco Pops™	77	30 g	26	20
Cornflakes™	77	30 g	25	20
Honey Rice Bubbles™	77	30 g	27	20
Oat 'n' Honey Bake™	77	30 g	17	13
Corn Pops™	80	30 g	26	21
Puffed Wheat	80	30 g	21	17
Rice Bubbles™	87	30 g	26	22
Cereal grains				
Pearl Barley, boiled	25	150 g	32	8
Rye, whole kernels	34	50 g	38	13
Wheat, whole kernels, cooked	41	50 g	34	14
Cracked wheat (bulghur), cooked	48*	150 g	26	12
Sweet corn	48	150 g	30	14

* Average

FOOD	GI	NOMINAL SERVE SIZE	AVAILABLE CARB PER SERVE	GL PER SERVE
Koshikari (Japanese) white rice, boiled	48	150 g	42	20
Parboiled, Doongara rice, boiled	50	150 g	39	19
Buckwheat, boiled	54	150 g	30	16
Wheat, quick-cooking kernels	54	150 g	47	25
Rice, brown, boiled	55	150 g	33	18
Semolina, cooked	55	150 g	11	6
Doongara rice, white	56	150 g	39	22
Long grain rice, boiled	56	150 g	41	23
Basmati rice, boiled (Mahatma, Australia)	58	150 g	38	22
Couscous	65	150 g	33	21
Barley, rolled	66	50 g	38	25
Doongara rice, brown, boiled	66	150 g	37	24
Arborio, risotto rice, boiled	69	150 g	53	36
Cornmeal, boiled	69	150 g	13	9
Pelde brown rice, boiled	76	150 g	38	29
Sunbrown rice Quick™, boiled	80	150 g	38	31
Calrose rice, white, medium grain, boiled	83	150 g	43	36
Calrose rice, brown, boiled	87	150 g	38	33
Instant rice, white, cooked 6 min	87	150 g	42	36
Parboiled rice, Sungold	87	150 g	39	34
Sungold rice, Pelde, parboiled	87	150 g	43	37
Pelde, white	93	150 g	43	40
Instant Doongara rice, white	94	150 g	42	35
Jasmine rice	109	150 g	42	46
Crackers				
Jatz™	55	25 g	17	10
Vita-wheat™, original, crispbread	55	25 g	19	10
Rye crispbread	64*	25 g	16	11

* Average

FOOD	GI	NOMINAL SERVE SIZE	AVAILABLE CARB PER SERVE	GL PER SERVE
Breton wheat crackers	67	25 g	14	10
Sao™, plain square crackers	70	25 g	17	12
Kavli™ Norwegian Crispbread	71	25 g	16	12
Water cracker	78	25 g	18	14
Puffed Crispbread	81	25 g	19	15
Puffed rice cakes	82	25 g	21	17
Dairy products				
Yoghurt, low fat, fruit, aspartame, Ski™	14	200 g	13	2
Milk, low fat, chocolate, no added sugar	24	250 ml	15	3
Milk, full-fat, fresh	31	250 ml	12	4
Yoghurt, low fat, fruit, sugar, Ski™	33	200 g	31	10
Mousse, reduced fat, from mix	34*	50 g	10	4
Ice-cream, Prestige Light™, traditional toffee (Norco, Australia)	37	50 g	14	5
Ice-cream, Ultra chocolate, 15% fat (Sara Lee, Australia)	37	50 g	9	4
Ice-cream, Prestige™, golden macadamia (Norco, Australia)	37	50 g	9	3
Custard	38*	100 g	16	6
Ice-cream, French vanilla, 16% fat (Sara Lee, Australia)	38	50 g	9	3
Reduced-fat yoghurt drink, Vaalia™, passionfruit	38	200 g	29	11
Yoghurt, no-fat, Strawberry, Vaalia, with sugar	38	150 ml	22	8
Yoghurt, no-fat, Wildberry, Vaalia, with sugar	38	150 ml	22	8

* Average

FOOD	GI	NOMINAL SERVE SIZE	AVAILABLE CARB PER SERVE	GL PER SERVE
Yoghurt, no-fat, Mango, Vaalia, with sugar	39	150 ml	25	10
Yoghurt, no-fat, French Vanilla, Vaalia, with sugar	40	150 ml	27	10
Milk, chocolate, sugar-sweetened	43	50 ml	28	12
Ice-cream, vanilla, Peter's Light and Creamy	44	150 ml	13	6
Ice-cream, vanilla, Prestige Light™ (Norco, Australia)	47	50 g	10	5
Ice-cream, vanilla	50	50 g	6	3
Ice-cream, regular	61	50 g	13	8
Fruit				
Cherries	22	120 g	12	3
Grapefruit	25	120 g	11	3
Pear halves, canned in reduced-sugar syrup (SPC Lite)	25	120 g	14	4
Apple, dried	29	60 g	34	10
Prunes, pitted	29	60 g	33	10
Apricots, dried	31*	60 g	27	8
Peach, canned in natural juice	38	120 g	11	4
Apple	38*	120 g	15	6
Pears	38	120 g	11	4
Plum	3*	120 g	12	5
Strawberries	40	120 g	3	1
Oranges	42	120 g	11	5
Peach	42*	120 g	8	5
Pear halves, canned in natural juice	43	120 g	13	5
Grapes	46*	120 g	18	8
Mango	51*	120 g	15	8
Banana	52*	120 g	26	13

* Average

FOOD	GI	NOMINAL SERVE SIZE	AVAILABLE CARB PER SERVE	GL PER SERVE
Kiwi fruit	53*	120 g	12	6
Sultanas	56	60 g	45	25
Grapes, black	59	120 g	18	11
Paw paw	56	120 g	8	5
Pineapple	59*	120 g	13	7
Figs	61	60 g	26	16
Raisins	64	60 g	44	28
Rockmelon	65	120 g	6	4
Watermelon	72	120 g	6	4
Lychee, canned in syrup, drained	79	120 g	20	16
Dates, dried	103	60 g	40	42
Fruit juice				
Apple juice, pure, cloudy (Wild About Fruit, Australia)	37	250 ml	28	10
Tomato juice, canned	38	250 ml	9	4
Apple juice, unsweetened	40	250 ml	29	12
Carrot juice	43	250 ml	23	10
Apple juice, pure, clear (Wild About Fruit, Australia)	44	250 ml	30	13
Pineapple juice, unsweetened	46	250 ml	34	16
Grapefruit juice, unsweetened	48	250 ml	22	11
Cranberry juice cocktail	52	250 ml	31	16
Orange juice, unsweetened	50	250 ml	19	9
Legumes				
Soy beans, dried, boiled	18*	150 g	6	1
Peas, dried, boiled	22	150 g	9	2
Lentils, red, dried, boiled	26*	150 g	18	5
Chickpeas, dried, boiled	28*	150 g	24	7
Kidney beans, dried, cooked	28*	150 g	25	7
Lentils, boiled	29	150 g	18	5
Lentils, green, dried, boiled	30*	150 g	17	5

* Average

FOOD	GI	NOMINAL SERVE SIZE	AVAILABLE CARB PER SERVE	GL PER SERVE
Butter Beans, boiled	31*	150 g	20	6
Mung bean, dried, boiled	42	150 g	17	7
Lima beans, baby, cooked	32	150 g	30	10
Split peas, yellow, boiled	32	150 g	19	6
Haricot/navy beans, pressure cooked	38	150 g	31	12
Marrowfat peas	39	150 g	19	7
Blackeyed beans, boiled	42*	150 g	21	12
Baked Beans, canned	48*	150 g	15	7
Meat				
Beef	[0]	120 g	0	0
Lamb	[0]	120 g	0	0
Pork	[0]	120 g	0	0
Salami	[0]	120 g	0	0
Tuna	[0]	120 g	0	0
Veal	[0]	120 g	0	0
Pasta and noodles				
Spaghetti, wholemeal, boiled	37*	180 g	42	16
Mung bean noodles	39	180 g	45	18
Ravioli	39	180 g	38	15
Fettucine, egg, boiled	40	180 g	46	18
Rice noodles	40	180 g	39	15
Spaghetti, white, boiled	42*	180 g	47	20
Spirali, durum wheat, white, boiled	43	180 g	44	19
Spaghetti, white, boiled 10–15 min	44*	180 g	48	21
Instant noodles	47	180 g	40	19
Macaroni	47	180 g	48	23
Linguine	49*	180 g	47	23

* Average

FOOD	GI	NOMINAL SERVE SIZE	AVAILABLE CARB PER SERVE	GL PER SERVE
Spaghetti, white, boiled 20 min	61*	180 g	44	27
Udon noodles, plain	62	180 g	48	30
Macaroni and Cheese, boxed (Kraft, Canada)	64	180 g	51	32
Gnocchi	68	180 g	48	33
Spaghetti, gluten-free, canned in tomato sauce	68	220 g	27	19
Rice pasta, brown, boiled	92	180 g	38	35
Potato				
Yam	37	150 g	36	13
Sweet potato	44	150 g	25	11
Taro	55	150 g	8	4
Boiled potatoes, Ontario	58	150 g	27	16
Baked potato, Ontario	60	150 g	30	18
New potato	62	150 g	21	13
Canned potato, new	65	150 g	18	12
Potato, peeled, steamed	65	150 g	27	18
Swede	72	150 g	10	7
French fries	75	150 g	29	22
Pontiac, peeled and microwaved on high for 6–7.5 min	79	150 g	18	14
Baked, Russet Burbank potato	85	150 g	30	26
Instant mashed potato	85	150 g	20	17
Boiled potatoes, Sebago	87	150 g	17	14
Boiled potatoes, Pontiac	88	150 g	18	16
Mashed potato, Pontiac	91	150 g	20	18
Boiled potatoes, Desiree	101	150 g	17	17
Rice				
Parboiled rice, Doongara	50	150 g	39	19
Rice, brown	55	150 g	33	18
Doongara rice, white	56	150 g	39	22

* Average

FOOD	GI	NOMINAL SERVE SIZE	AVAILABLE CARB PER SERVE	GL PER SERVE
Long grain rice, boiled	56	150 g	41	23
Basmati rice, boiled	58	150 g	42	24
Doongara rice, brown	66	150 g	37	24
Arborio, risotto rice, boiled	69	150 g	43	29
Pelde rice, brown	76	150 g	38	29
Sunbrown Quick™ rice	80	150 g	38	31
Calrose rice, white, medium grain, boiled	83	150 g	42	35
Calrose rice brown	87	150 g	40	35
Instant rice, white	87	150 g	42	36
Parboiled rice, Sungold	87	150 g	39	34
Sungold rice, Pelde, parboiled	87	150 g	43	37
Pelde rice, white	93	150 g	43	40
Instant Doongara rice, white	94	150 g	42	35
Jasmine rice, long grain	109	150 g	42	46
Snacks				
M & M's®, peanut	33	30 g	17	6
Nutella®	33	20 g	12	4
Fruity Bitz	39*	15 g	12	4
Snickers Bar®	41	60 g	36	15
Corn chips, plain, salted	42	50 g	25	11
Chocolate, milk, plain	43*	50 g	28	12
Chocolate, white, Milky Bar®	44	50 g	29	13
Twix bar®	44	60 g	39	17
Apricot filled fruit bar	50	50 g	34	17
Potato crisps, plain, salted	57	50 g	18	10
Heinz Kidz™ Fruit Fingers	61	30 g	20	12
Muesli bar, with dried fruit	61	30 g	21	13
Mars Bar®	62	60 g	40	25
Life Savers®	70	30 g	30	21
Pop Tarts™, chocolate	70	50 g	35	24

* Average

FOOD	GI	NOMINAL SERVE SIZE	AVAILABLE CARB PER SERVE	GL PER SERVE
Skittles®	70	50 g	45	32
Popcorn, cooked in microwave	72	20 g	11	8
Twisties™	74	50 g	29	22
Jelly beans	78	30 g	28	22
Pretzels, oven baked	83	30 g	20	16
Burger Rings™	90	50 g	31	28
Real Fruit Bars™, strawberry	90	30 g	26	23
Roll-Ups®	99	30 g	25	24
Soft drinks				
Coca Cola®, soft drink	53	250 ml	26	14
Solo™, lemon squash, soft drink	58	250 ml	29	17
Cordial, orange	66	250 ml	20	13
Fanta®, orange soft drink	68	250 ml	34	23
Lucozade®, original	95	250 ml	42	40
Soups				
Tomato soup	38	250 ml	17	6
Minestrone, Country Ladle™	39	250 ml	18	7
Lentil, canned	44	250 ml	21	9
Split Pea	60	250 ml	27	16
Black Bean	64	250 ml	27	17
Green Pea, canned	66	250 ml	41	27
Sports drinks				
Sustagen Sport®	43	250 ml	49	21
Isostar®	70	250 ml	18	13
Sports Plus®	74	250 ml	17	13
Gatorade®	78	250 ml	15	12
Sugars				
Fructose	19	10 g	10	2
Yellow box honey	35	25 g	18	6
Stringy Bark honey	44	25 g	21	9
Lactose	46	10 g	10	5

* Average

FOOD	GI	NOMINAL SERVE SIZE	AVAILABLE CARB PER SERVE	GL PER SERVE
Red Gum honey	46	25 g	18	8
Iron Bark honey	48	25 g	15	7
Yapunya honey	52	25 g	17	9
Pure Capilano™ honey	58	25 g	21	12
Sucrose	68*	10 g	10	6
Commercial Blend honey	62	25 g	18	11
Salvation Jane honey	64	25 g	15	10
Commercial Blend honey	72	25 g	13	9
Glucose	100	10 g	10	10
Maltose	105	10 g	10	11
Vegetables				
Carrots, peeled, boiled	41*	80 g	5	2
Green peas, boiled	48	80 g	7	3
Corn on the cob, sweet, boiled	48*	80 g	16	8
Beetroot, canned	64	80 g	7	5
Broad beans, cooked	79	80 g	11	9
Parsnips	97	80 g	12	12
Artichokes	[0]	80 g	0	0
Avocado	[0]	80 g	0	0
Bokchoy	[0]	80 g	0	0
Broccoli	[0]	80 g	0	0
Cabbage	[0]	80 g	0	0
Capsicum	[0]	80 g	0	0
Cauliflower	[0]	80 g	0	0
Celery	[0]	80 g	0	0
Cucumber	[0]	80 g	0	0
French beans (runner beans)	[0]	80 g	0	0
Leafy vegetables (spinach, rocket etc)	[0]	80 g	0	0
Lettuce	[0]	80 g	0	0

* Average

About the authors

Professor Jennie Brand-Miller is a Professor of Human Nutrition in the Human Nutrition Unit, School of Molecular and Microbial Biosciences at the University of Sydney and President of the Nutrition Society of Australia. She has taught postgraduate students of nutrition and dietetics at the University of Sydney for over 24 years and currently leads a team of 12 research scientists. Her most recent book is the best-selling *The GI Factor*, recently updated and republished as *The New Glucose Revolution*.

Kaye Foster-Powell, an accredited practising dietitian with extensive experience in diabetes management. A graduate of the University of Sydney (B. Sc., Master of Nutrition & Dietetics) she has conducted research into the glycaemic index of foods and its practical applications over the last 15 years. Currently she is a dietitian with Wentworth Area Diabetes Services and provides consultancy on all aspects of the glycaemic index. Her most recent book is the best-selling *The GI Factor*, recently updated and republished as *The New Glucose Revolution*.

Dr Susanna Holt works closely with Professor Jennie Brand-Miller as the Research Manager of Sydney University's Glycaemic Index Research Service (SUGiRS). Susanna is also a qualified dietitian and nutrition consultant.